Assessment of Sexual Maturity Stages in Girls and Boys

Marcia E. Herman-Giddens, PA, DrPH
Carlos J. Bourdony, MD, FAAP
Steven A. Dowshen, MD, FAAP
Edward O. Reiter, MD, FAAP

Pediatric Research in Office Settings
Department of Research

American Academy of Pediatrics
345 Park Blvd
Itasca, IL 60143

American Academy of Pediatrics Department of Marketing and Publications Staff

Maureen DeRosa, MPA
Director, Department of Marketing and Publications

Sandi King, MS
Director, Division of Publishing and Production Services

Jason Crase
Editorial Specialist

Leesa Levin-Doroba
Manager, Publishing and Production Services

Linda Diamond
Manager, Art Direction and Production

Linda Smessaert
Manager, Clinical and Professional Publications Marketing

ISBN: 978-1-58110-443-1
MA0544
11-73/rev0920

The recommendations in this publication do not indicate an exclusive course of treatment or serve as a standard of medical care. Variations, taking into account individual circumstances, may be appropriate.

This publication has been developed by the American Academy of Pediatrics. The authors, editors, and contributors are expert authorities in the field of pediatrics. No commercial involvement of any kind has been solicited or accepted in the development of the content of this publication.

Copyright © 2021 by the American Academy of Pediatrics. All rights reserved. No part of this publication may be reproduced, stored in a retrieval system, or transmitted in any form or by any means, electronic, mechanical, photocopying, recording, or otherwise, without prior written permission from the publisher. Printed in the United States of America.

Authors/Principal Investigators

Marcia E. Herman-Giddens, PA, DrPH

Marcia E. Herman-Giddens is a consultant in the areas of normal puberty and child maltreatment. After 3 years as the medical director of the North Carolina State Child Fatality Prevention Team, and 5 years as a Senior Fellow at the North Carolina Child Advocacy Institute (now known as Action for Children North Carolina), she has been engaged primarily in child advocacy, teaching, and research. She is an adjunct professor in the UNC Gillings School of Global Public Health, Department of Maternal and Child Health, University of North Carolina at Chapel Hill. She has worked in the field of child health and maltreatment for more than 25 years as a medical provider, advocate, teacher, and researcher. Her research, published in numerous journals, books, and monographs, has revolved around the growth and development of children, puberty, child sexual abuse, and child fatalities, especially those from abuse. Dr Herman-Giddens received her Physician Associate degree from Duke University Medical Center in 1978 and practiced pediatrics there for many years as well as directing its Child Protection Team. She received her doctorate in public health in 1994. She was the principal investigator of the seminal study of puberty in US girls conducted by Pediatric Research in Office Settings (PROS), American Academy of Pediatrics (AAP), and coauthor of *Assessment of Sexual Maturity Stages in Girls* (1995) and *Assessment of Sexual Maturity Stages in Boys* (2005).

Carlos J. Bourdony, MD, FAAP

Dr Bourdony received his medical degree from Mexico's National University School of Medicine and did his general pediatrics specialty and pediatric endocrinology and diabetes subspecialty at St. Christopher's Hospital for Children at Temple University in Philadelphia, PA. Currently, he is a principal investigator at the Latin Clinical Trial Center and board certified in pediatrics and pediatric endocrinology and diabetes with a private practice in San Juan, PR. Dr Bourdony is former director of the Department of Pediatric Endocrinology, San Juan City Hospital, San Juan, Puerto Rico. He was the founder, director, and medical advisor of the Puerto Rico Department of Health Premature Thelarche and Sexual Development Registry. He is also past president and current member of the Puerto Rico Society of Endocrinology and Diabetes. Dr Bourdony has done extensive research in the area of premature thelarche in Puerto Rican girls. He was a coinvestigator of the seminal study of puberty in US girls conducted by PROS, AAP, and coauthor of *Assessment of Sexual Maturity Stages in Girls* (1995).

Steven A. Dowshen, MD, FAAP

Dr Dowshen was a board-certified pediatrician and subspecialist in pediatric endocrinology practicing at Alfred I. duPont Hospital for Children in Wilmington, DE. He received his BS from Pennsylvania State University and his MD from Jefferson Medical College of Thomas Jefferson University, and completed his pediatric residency and fellowship training in pediatric endocrinology and metabolism at St. Christopher's Hospital for Children in Philadelphia, PA. He was chief medical editor of the Nemours Foundation Center for Children's Health Media and KidsHealth.org, the most visited site on the Web providing consumer health information for parents, children, and teens. Dr Dowshen was director of the Nemours Fellowship in Children's Health Media, a chapter officer and the PROS coordinator for the Delaware Chapter of the AAP, a member of the Lawson Wilkins Pediatric Endocrine Society, and chairman of Kids Count in Delaware. Prior to joining the staff at Alfred I. duPont Hospital for Children, Dr Dowshen was director of the pediatric residency training program at the Albert Einstein Medical Center in Philadelphia.

Edward O. Reiter, MD, FAAP

A graduate of Rutgers University and the University of Rochester School of Medicine and Dentistry, Dr Reiter had residency training at Rainbow Babies & Children's Hospital in Cleveland, OH, and the University of California, San Francisco. He was a Pediatric Endocrinology Fellow at the National Institutes of Health and at the University of California, San Francisco. Subsequently, he was on the faculty at the University of South Florida, and then moved to Massachusetts in 1978, becoming chairman of the Department of Pediatrics at Baystate Medical Center in 1982 and professor of pediatrics at Tufts University School of Medicine. Dr Reiter's research interest is in the area of the endocrine control of childhood growth and pubertal maturation. He is a board-certified (and recertified) pediatric endocrinologist. He has more than 170 publications and 70 abstracts, and has delivered many invited lectureships. Dr Reiter is a member of the Lawson Wilkins Pediatric Endocrine Society, American Pediatric Society/Society for Pediatric Research, Endocrine Society, and the AAP. He was the president of the Lawson Wilkins Pediatric Endocrine Society in 2000–2001.

Table of Contents

vii	Foreword
viii	Acknowledgments

1 Assessment of Sexual Maturity Stages in Girls

3	Introduction
4	Breast Maturity Ratings: The Tanner Photographs
5	Pubic Hair Ratings: The Tanner Photographs
6	Breast Maturity Ratings: The van Wieringen Photographs
7	Pubic Hair Ratings: The van Wieringen Photographs
8	Staging Breast Development
13	Staging Pubic Hair Development
15	Staging Axillary Hair Development
16	Examination Techniques
17	The Influence of Breast Types on Assessment of Stage of Development
18	Assignment of Stages for Breast and Pubic Hair Development

19 Assessment of Sexual Maturity Stages in Boys

21	Introduction
22	Genital Maturity Ratings: The Tanner Photographs
23	Genital Maturity Ratings: The van Wieringen Photographs
24	Staging Genital Development
27	Staging Pubic Hair Growth
29	Examples of Subtleties of Staging
31	Staging Axillary Hair Development
32	Examination Techniques
37	References

Foreword

Age of onset of pubertal characteristics is important for medical, social, and public health reasons. In the last 20 years there has been a renewed interest worldwide in pubertal data due to many countries finding that, contrary to earlier studies, the age of pubertal markers was continuing to decline, though at a much slower rate than in the first half of the 20th century. In addition, it is now recognized that important racial and ethnic differences exist as well. Knowing how to accurately assess sexual maturity markers is an important clinical skill.

Secular changes in ages of onset of pubertal markers have profound public health implications. Just as rising ages may indicate harmful social or environmental conditions including inadequate nutrition, lowering ages may not indicate ideal health but may reflect undesirable factors. For example, many recent studies have demonstrated the association between the epidemic of overweight and obese girls and earlier pubertal onset and menarche. Questions about interactions between overweight and puberty in boys await more studies for clarity. Endocrine disrupters are increasingly found to be associated with early and late puberty depending on the chemical and sex of the child. Many other factors, including prenatal conditions, are also being studied for their associations with pubertal age.

Observation of the development of genital and sexual hair growth in children is an essential part of their physical examination. Accurate staging of the physical changes of sexual development provides an important basis for the diagnosis and management of certain clinical problems that may arise as the child grows and matures. In addition, counseling of patients and families regarding the expected timing and sequence of pubertal development depends on accurate physical assessment and understanding of the stages of development.

This manual is a combination and revision from those developed for the Pediatric Research in Office Settings (PROS) puberty study on girls in 1995[1] and for the PROS puberty study on boys in 2005.[2] It will assist you in learning how to assign the stages of the physical changes of pubertal development using the systems described by Marshall and Tanner[3,4] as well as correct techniques for breast palpation and testicular measurement. Because gynecomastia is common among and of concern to adolescent boys, assessing breast tissue is important for boys as well as girls.

Photographs

The 2 "classic" sets of photographs of the 5 male and female sexual maturity stages in medical literature are those of Tanner[5] and van Wieringen et al.[6] This manual uses these classic photographs as well as many taken for this book. Drawings for each genital and pubic hair stage with further explanatory detail are also included to supplement the photographs.

Acknowledgments

The Assessment of Sexual Maturity Stages in Girls section was developed as a part of a larger project conducted by the Pediatric Research in Office Settings (PROS) network. PROS, a primary care research network, is a program of the American Academy of Pediatrics (AAP) Department of Research.

The project, a prevalence study of secondary sexual characteristics of young girls seen in office practice, was originally funded by Genentech, Inc, the US Maternal and Child Health Bureau, and the AAP.

The development of the manual was also assisted by Duke University Medical Center Department of Pediatrics and the Audiovisual Education Department, the San Juan City Hospital, and the University of Puerto Rico School of Medicine Division of Educational Technology.

The assistance of James M. Tanner, MD, PhD; Ana M. Lugo, RN, San Juan City Hospital; the staff of the Audiovisual Education Department of Duke University Medical Center; and the children who participated is gratefully acknowledged.

The Assessment of Sexual Maturity Stages in Boys section was developed as part of a larger project conducted by the PROS network called *Secondary Sexual Characteristics in Boys*. The project, a prevalence study of secondary sexual characteristics of young boys seen in office practice, was funded by the Genentech Center for Clinical Research in Endocrinology; the Georgia Health Foundation; the AAP; the Health Resources and Services Administration, Maternal and Child Health Bureau; and Pfizer. The principal investigators are Marcia E. Herman-Giddens, PA, DrPH, and Edward O. Reiter, MD, FAAP.

We are grateful to Marsha L. Davenport, MD, professor of pediatrics, Division of Pediatric Endocrinology, Department of Pediatrics, University of North Carolina School of Medicine, Chapel Hill, who provided photographs for the use of the orchidometer; John S. Fuqua, MD, associate professor of clinical pediatrics, Section of Pediatric Endocrinology and Diabetology, Department of Pediatrics, Indiana University School of Medicine and Riley Hospital for Children, Indianapolis, who provided photographs demonstrating certain aspects of Tanner Staging of boys; and Medical Illustrations, University of North Carolina School of Medicine, Chapel Hill, for its photography work. We are also grateful to Stanley Coffman from the Duke University School of Medicine Department of Educational Media Services in Durham, NC, for providing the drawings and to John Fuqua, MD, for providing additional photographs, reviewing the manual, and providing expert suggestions. In addition, we would like to acknowledge Paul Kaplowitz, MD, Children's National Medical Center, Washington, DC; Reuben Rohn, MD, Children's Hospital of the King's Daughters, Norfolk, VA; and Susan Rose, MD, Cincinnati Children's Hospital Medical Center, for reviewing the manual and providing expert suggestions.

We wish to acknowledge the following AAP staff for their excellence in project management and editing expertise: Kathy Thoma, MA; Alison Bocian, MS; Jennifer Steffes, MSW; Donna Harris, MA; and Eric Slora, PhD.

Assessment of Sexual Maturity Stages in Girls

Introduction

Determining the degree of development of the breasts and pubic and axillary hair in girls is an essential part of the physical examination. Accurate staging provides an important basis for the management of certain clinical problems that may arise as the child grows. In addition, counseling regarding the expected timing and sequence of pubertal development depends on recording and understanding the stages of development.

The following material demonstrates how to assign the stages of secondary sexual development using the system described by Tanner.[7]

Sexual Maturity Ratings

The system of sexual maturity rating presented in this manual is based on the work of Marshall and Tanner.[3,4,7] This rating system has been used widely in studies around the world.[8–16] Staging of sexual development was first described by Stratz in 1901 and included 4 maturity ratings for the breast.[17] Reynolds and Wines added the fifth breast stage as part of their longitudinal study in the 1940s, which was then adapted by Marshall and Tanner.[18]

It is helpful for examiners to be familiar with the classic sets of pubertal photographs. Because these sets lack details important for assessing certain features of sexual maturity, photographs or drawings produced for this manual of each breast, pubic, and axillary stage are also included.

Breast Palpation

Breast palpation is not part of Tanner staging. With the rise of the prevalence of overweight children, it is harder to determine true breast development by visual inspection. Therefore, accurate assessments of breast development or the presence of gynecomastia may require palpation.

It is important to note that there are no breast tissue sizes that correspond with specific Tanner stages with the exception of the breast "bud" in females. The use of palpation should be recorded in the clinical note and should not influence the visual assessment of stage.

The terms used in describing sexual maturity stages are as follows:

Definitions

Areola: the circular, darkly pigmented area of the skin surrounding the nipple

Mons: the rounded, fleshy prominence over the symphysis pubis

Papilla: the pigmented projection on the breast surrounded by the areola; also called the nipple

Pubis: the pubic bone, the junction of the anterior portion of the hip bones

Vellus: the fine hair that succeeds the lanugo over most of the body and persists until puberty

Breast Maturity Ratings: The Tanner Photographs

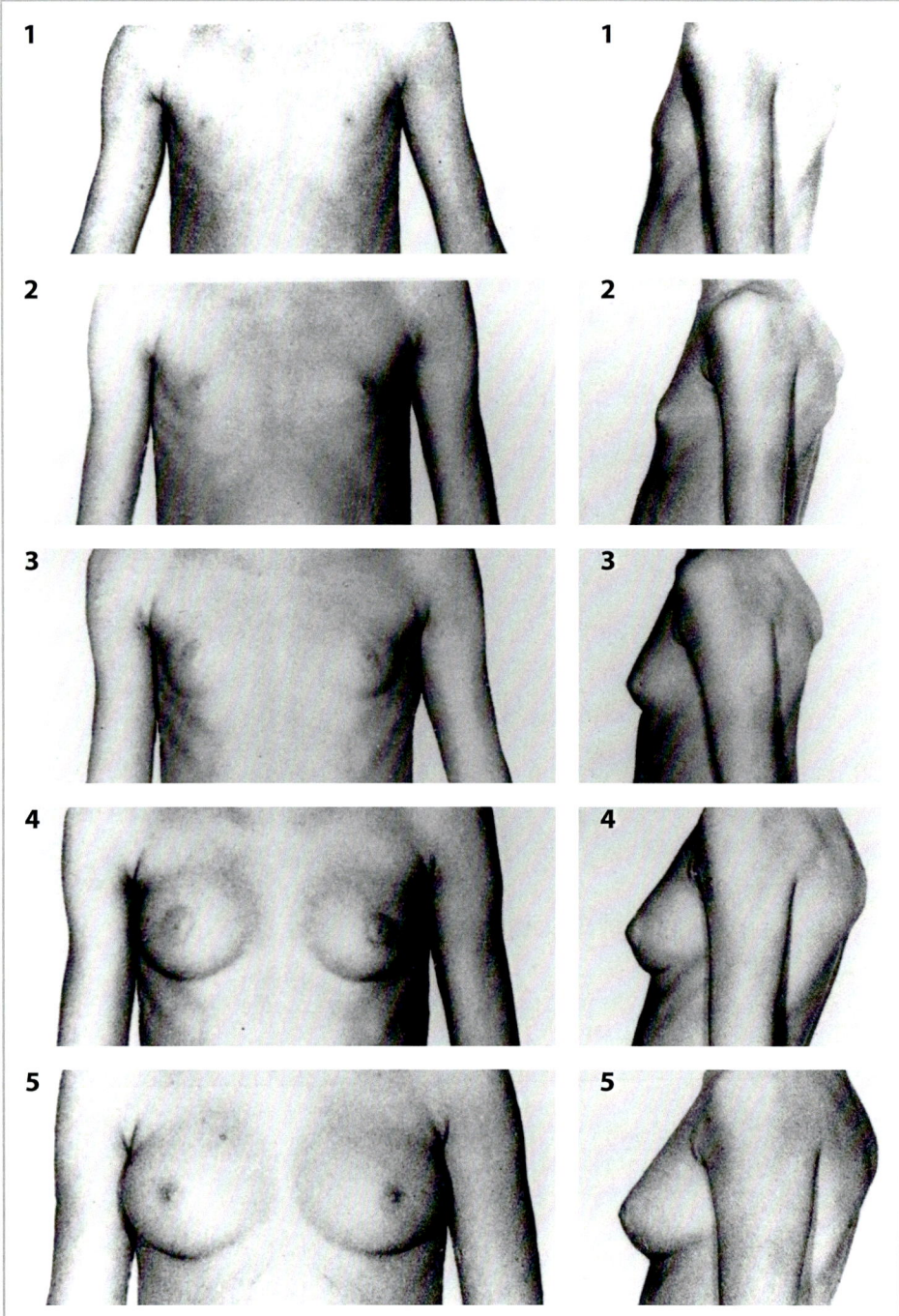

Breast Stage 1 (B$_1$)
The infantile stage, which persists from the postnatal period until the onset of puberty.

Breast Stage 2 (B$_2$)
The "bud" stage. The breast and papilla are elevated as a small mound. The diameter of the areola is increased.

Breast Stage 3 (B$_3$)
The breast and areola are further enlarged with a continuous rounded contour.

Breast Stage 4 (B$_4$)
The areola and papilla continue to expand and form a secondary mound projecting above the contour of the breast.

Breast Stage 5 (B$_5$)
The adult form with a smooth rounded contour. The secondary mound present in Stage 4 is gone.

SOURCE: Tanner JM. *Growth at Adolescence.* 2nd ed. Oxford, UK: Blackwell Scientific Publications; 1962. Reproduced with permission of Blackwell Publishing Ltd.

Pubic Hair Ratings: The Tanner Photographs

Pubic Hair Stage 1 (PH₁)
None

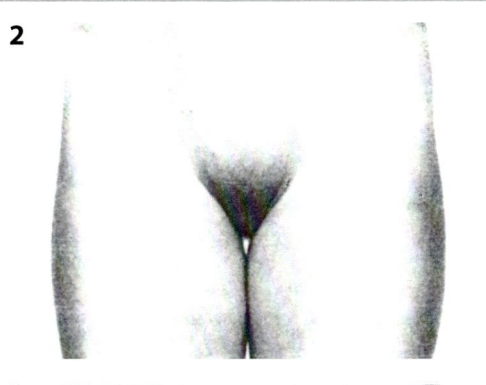

Pubic Hair Stage 2 (PH₂)
Small amount of long, downy hair along the labia majora.*

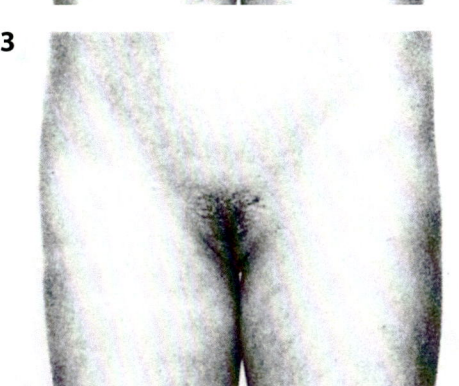

Pubic Hair Stage 3 (PH₃)
Moderate amount of more curly, pigmented, and coarser hair. The hair also beings to extend laterally.

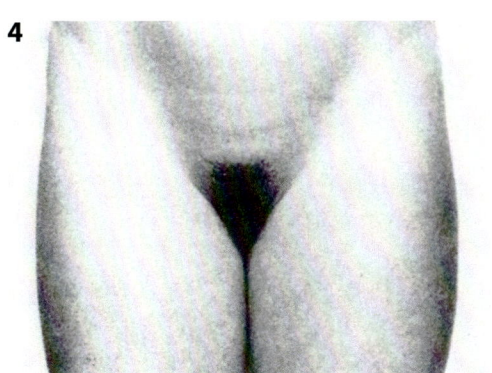

Pubic Hair Stage 4 (PH₄)
Hair that resembles adult hair in coarseness and curliness, but area covered is smaller and there is no extension to the medial surface of thighs.

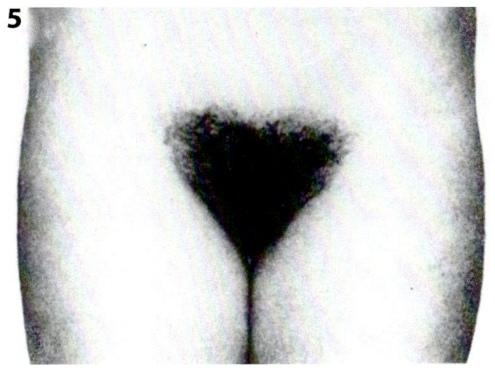

Pubic Hair Stage 5 (PH₅)
Adult type and quantity, sometimes extending to medial surface of thighs.

SOURCE: Tanner JM. *Growth at Adolescence.* 2nd ed. Oxford, UK: Blackwell Scientific Publications; 1962. Reproduced with permission of Blackwell Publishing Ltd.

*The shadow in this photograph obscures the detail of this stage.

Breast Maturity Ratings: The van Wieringen Photographs

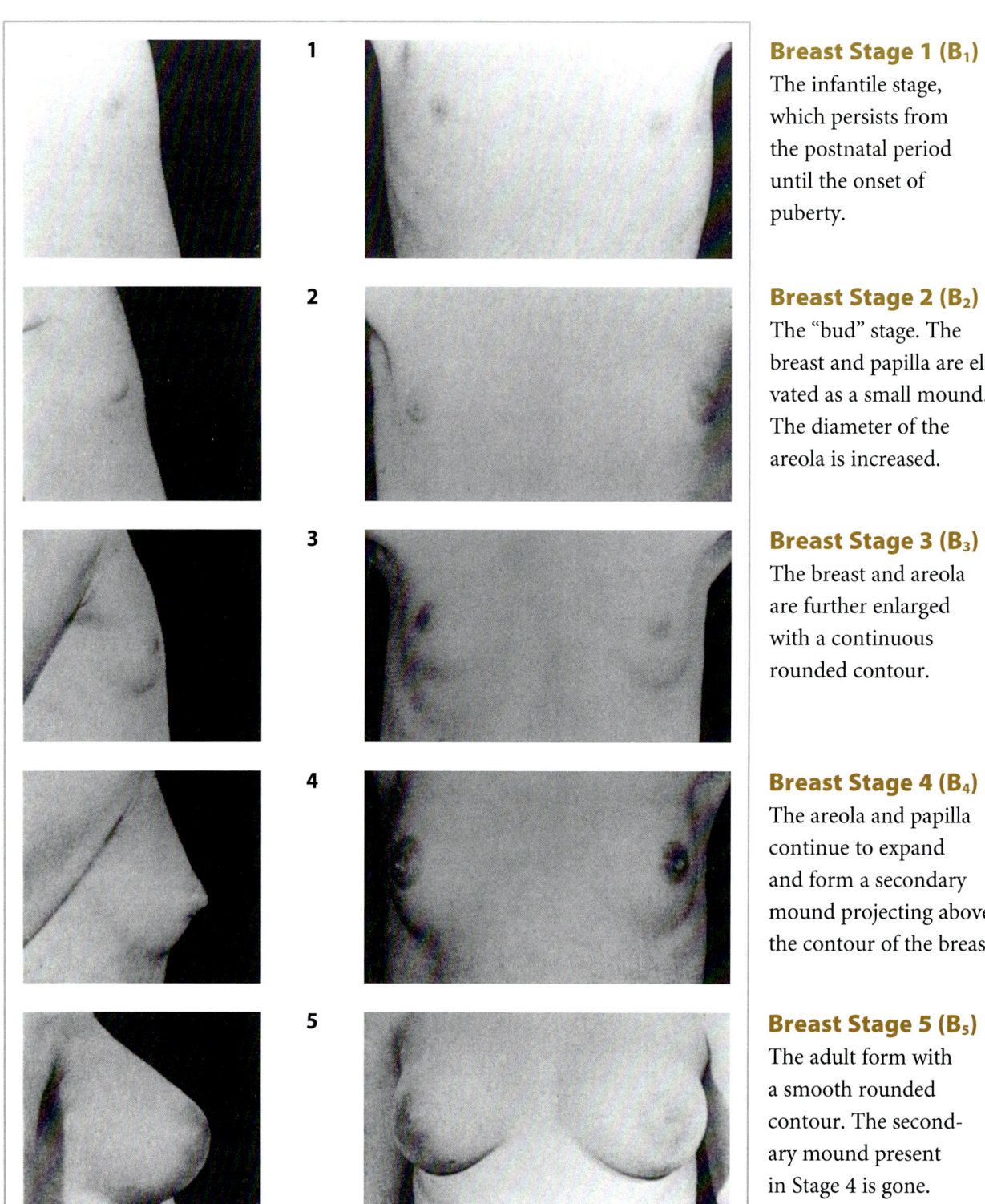

Breast Stage 1 (B$_1$)
The infantile stage, which persists from the postnatal period until the onset of puberty.

Breast Stage 2 (B$_2$)
The "bud" stage. The breast and papilla are elevated as a small mound. The diameter of the areola is increased.

Breast Stage 3 (B$_3$)
The breast and areola are further enlarged with a continuous rounded contour.

Breast Stage 4 (B$_4$)
The areola and papilla continue to expand and form a secondary mound projecting above the contour of the breast.

Breast Stage 5 (B$_5$)
The adult form with a smooth rounded contour. The secondary mound present in Stage 4 is gone.

SOURCE: Reprinted by permission from van Wieringen JC, Wafelbakker F, Verbrugge HP, De Haas JH. *Growth Diagrams 1965.* Groningen, The Netherlands: Wolters-Noordhoff; 1971. As included in Yen SSC, Jaffe RB (eds): *Reproductive Endocrinology: Physiology, Pathophysiology and Clinical Management,* 2nd ed. Philadelphia, PA: WB Saunders; 1978. Copyright Elsevier.

Pubic Hair Ratings: The van Wieringen Photographs

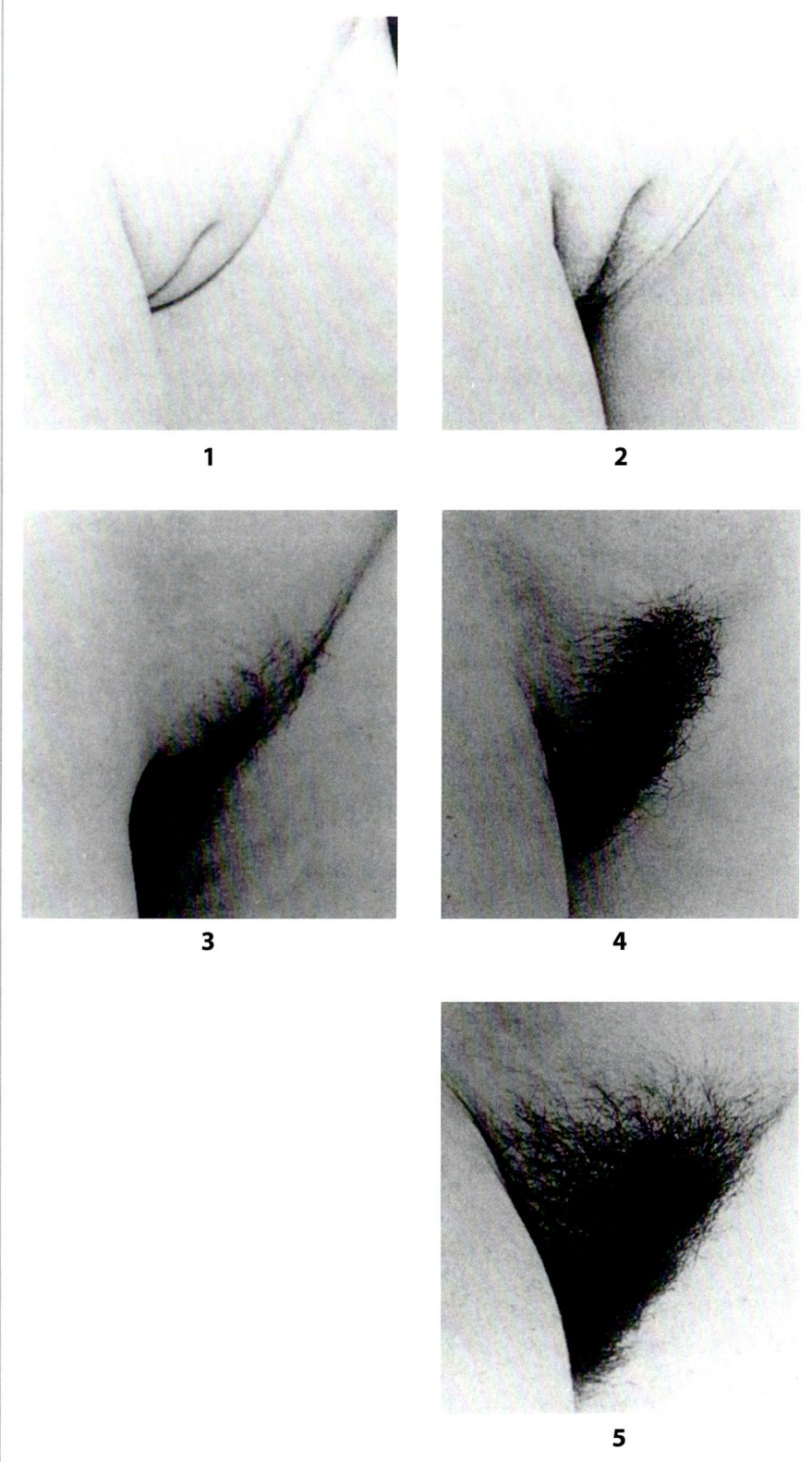

Pubic Hair Stage 1 (PH$_1$)
None.

Pubic Hair Stage 2 (PH$_2$)
Small amount of long, downy hair along the labia majora.

Pubic Hair Stage 3 (PH$_3$)
Moderate amount of more curly, pigmented, and coarser hair. The hair also beings to extend laterally.

Pubic Hair Stage 4 (PH$_4$)
Hair that resembles adult hair in coarseness and curliness, but area covered is smaller and there is no extension to the medial surface of thighs.

Pubic Hair Stage 5 (PH$_5$)
Adult type and quantity, sometimes extending to medial surface of thighs.

SOURCE: Reprinted by permission from van Wieringen JC, Wafelbakker F, Verbrugge HP, De Haas JH. *Growth Diagrams 1965.* Groningen, The Netherlands: Wolters-Noordhoff; 1971. As included in Yen SSC, Jaffe RB (eds): *Reproductive Endocrinology: Physiology, Pathophysiology and Clinical Management,* 2nd ed. Philadelphia, PA: WB Saunders; 1978. Copyright Elsevier.

Staging Breast Development

The following descriptions, drawings, and photographs should be studied together.

Staging Breast Development
Assignment of stages is based on visual inspection only, as described by Marshall and Tanner.[3]

Breast Stage 1
There is no development. Only the papilla is elevated.

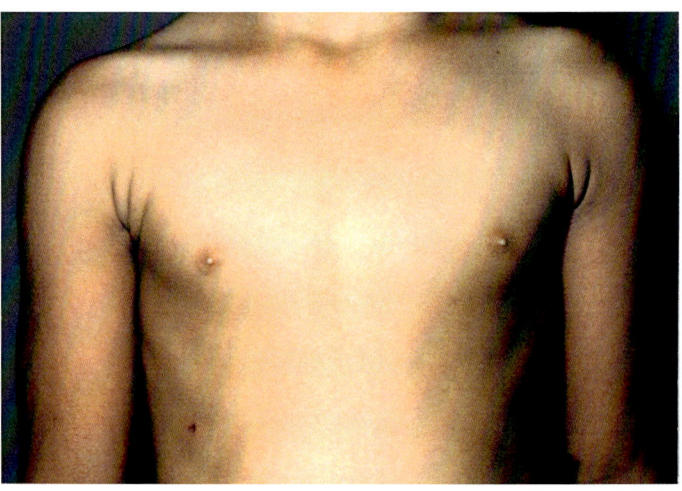

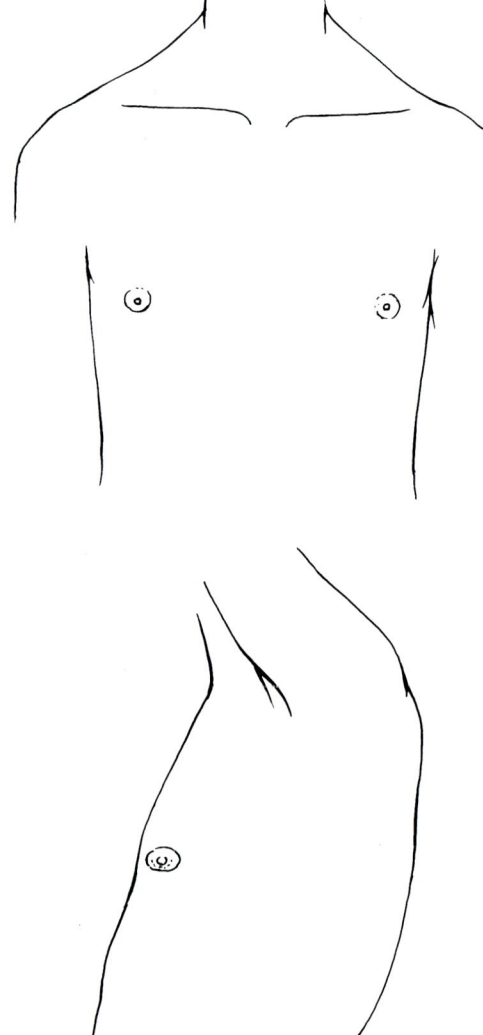

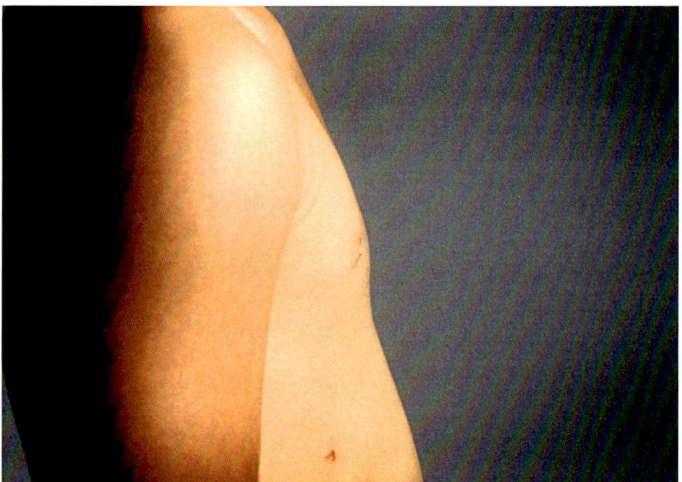

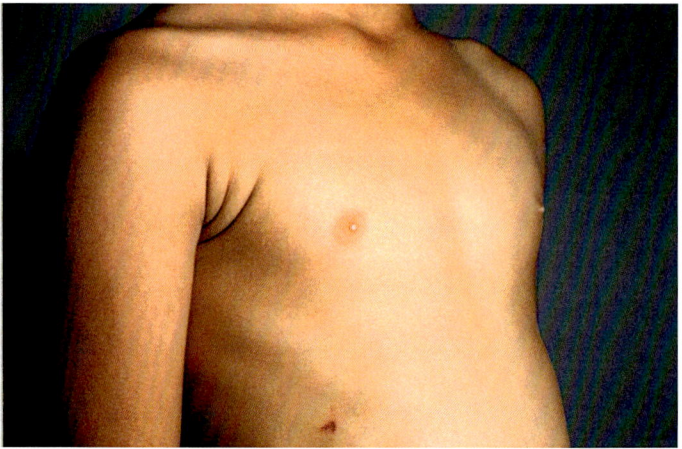

SOURCE: Carlos J. Bourdony, MD, former Director of Pediatric Endocrinology, San Juan City Hospital, San Juan, Puerto Rico.

Breast Stage 2

The "breast bud" stage. The areola widens, darkens slightly, and elevates from the rest of the breast as a small mound. A bud of breast tissue is palpable below the nipple.

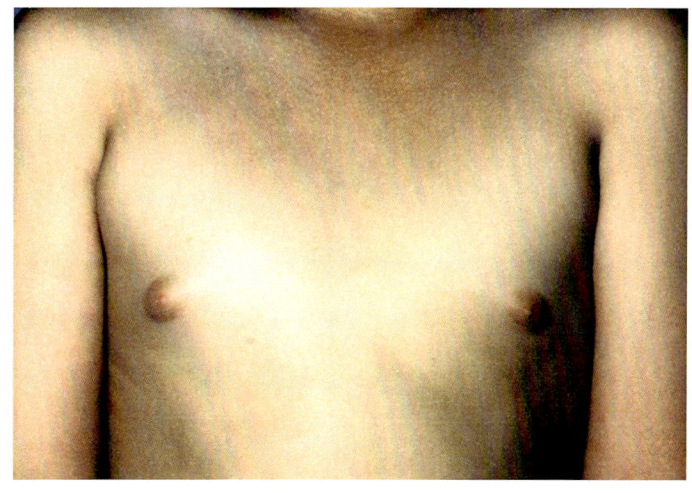

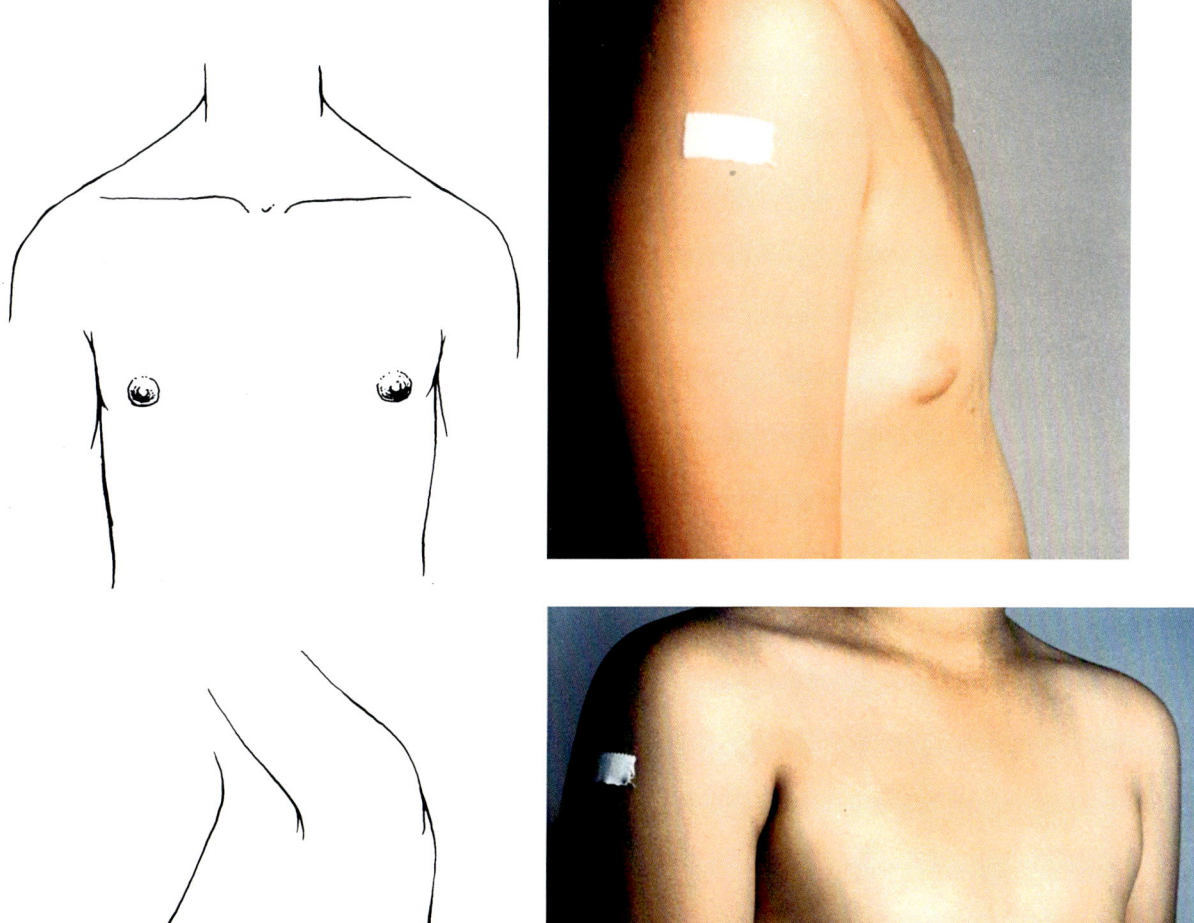

SOURCE: Carlos J. Bourdony, MD, former Director of Pediatric Endocrinology, San Juan City Hospital, San Juan, Puerto Rico.

Breast Stage 3

The breast and areola further enlarge and present a rounded contour. There is no separation of contour between the nipple and areola and the rest of the breast. Note that lack of separation of contour between the areola and the rest of the breast is also a feature of Stage 5. These stages may be distinguished from one another—even in a small-breasted individual—by the greater diameter of breast tissue in Stage 5. At Stage 3 the breast tissue creates a small cone, as opposed to the wider cone in Stage 5.

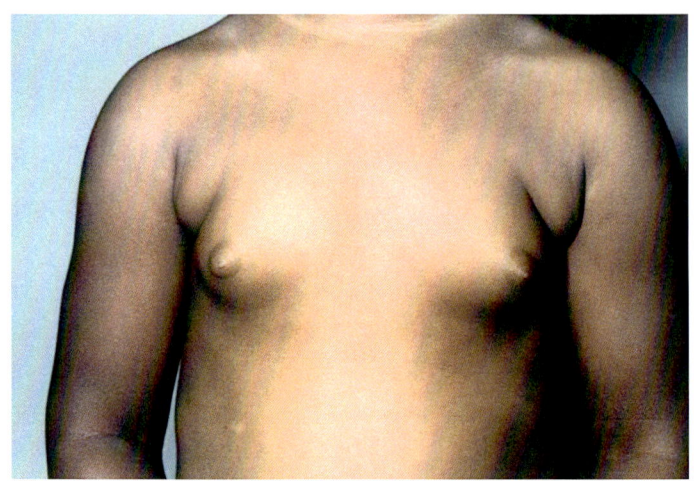
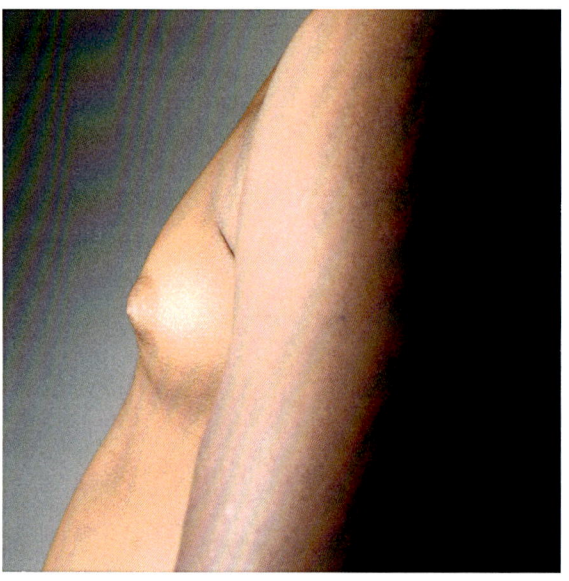
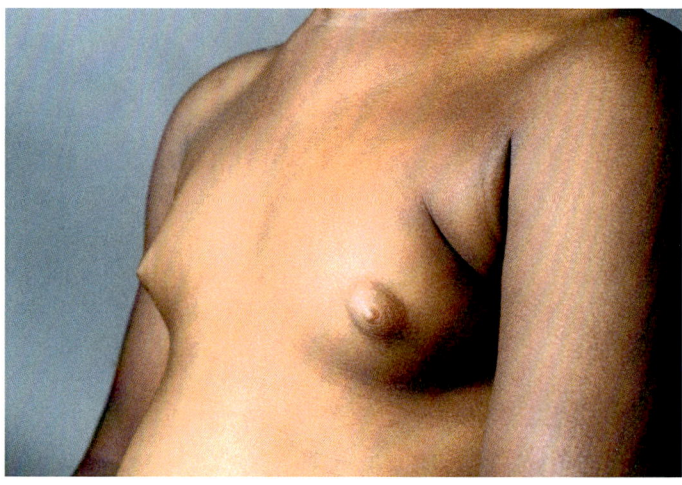
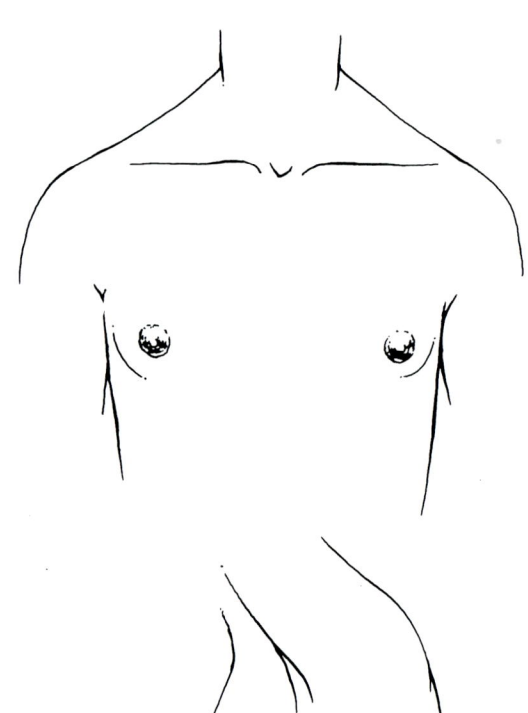

SOURCE: Carlos J. Bourdony, MD, former Director of Pediatric Endocrinology, San Juan City Hospital, San Juan, Puerto Rico.

Breast Stage 4

The breast continues to expand. The papilla and areola project to form a secondary mound above the rest of the breast tissue. Note depiction in drawing.

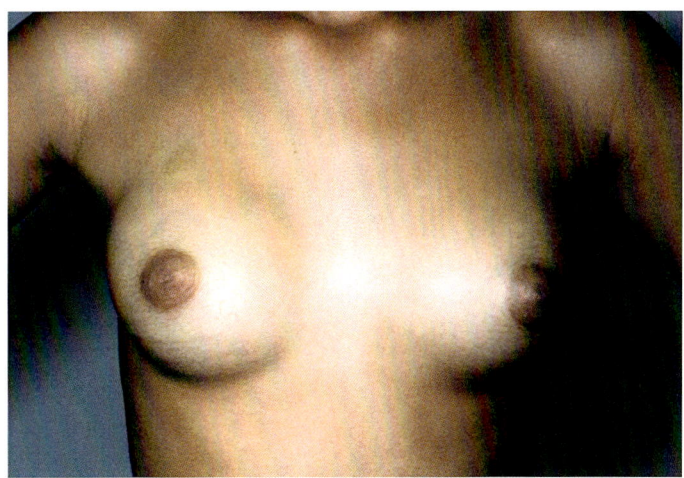

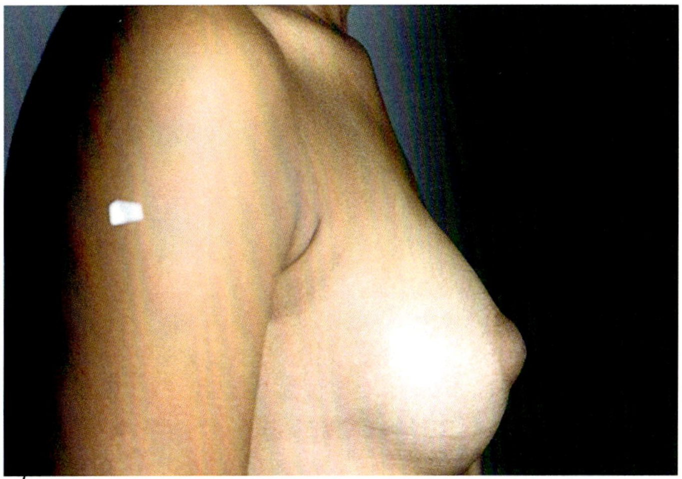

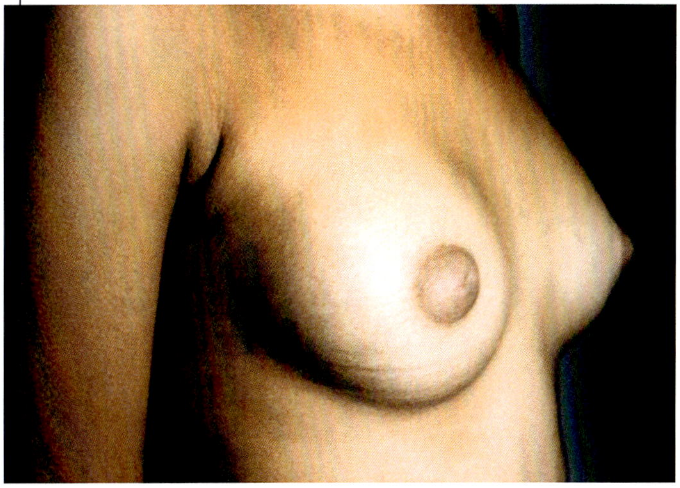

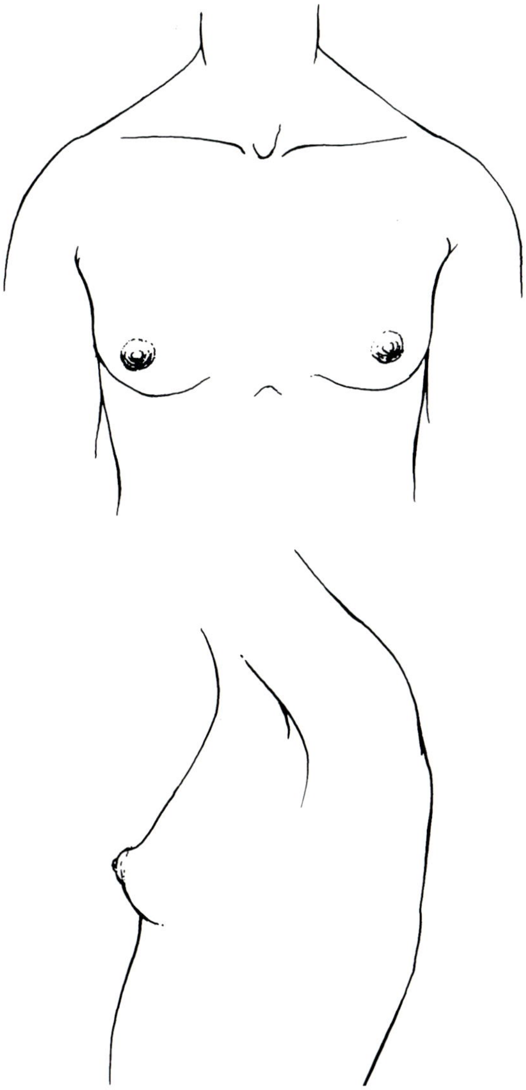

SOURCE: Carlos J. Bourdony, MD, former Director of Pediatric Endocrinology, San Juan City Hospital, San Juan, Puerto Rico.

Breast Stage 5

The mature adult stage. The secondary mound made by the areola and nipple present in Stage 4 disappears. Only the papilla projects. Even in a small-breasted individual, the diameter of the breast tissue (as opposed to the height) has extended to cover most of the area between the sternum and lateral chest wall.

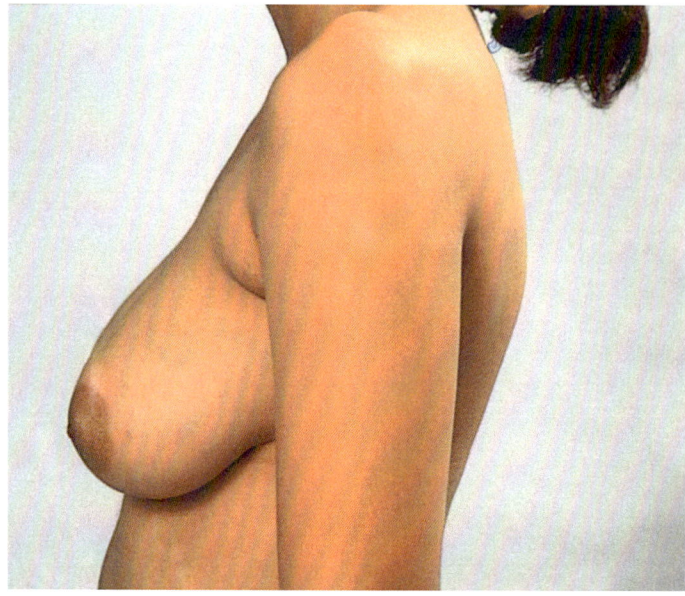
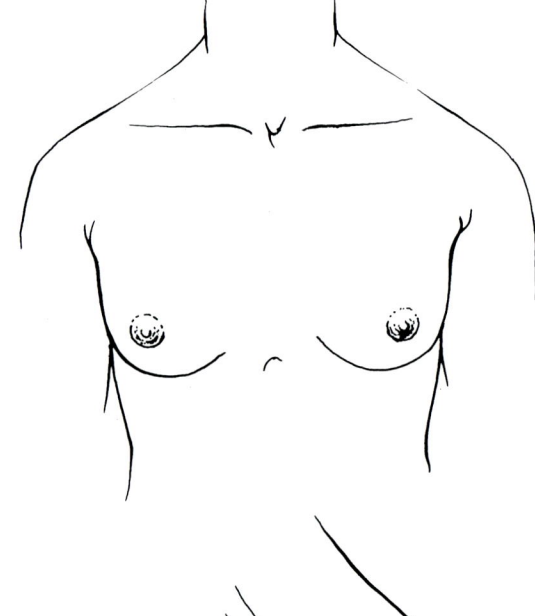
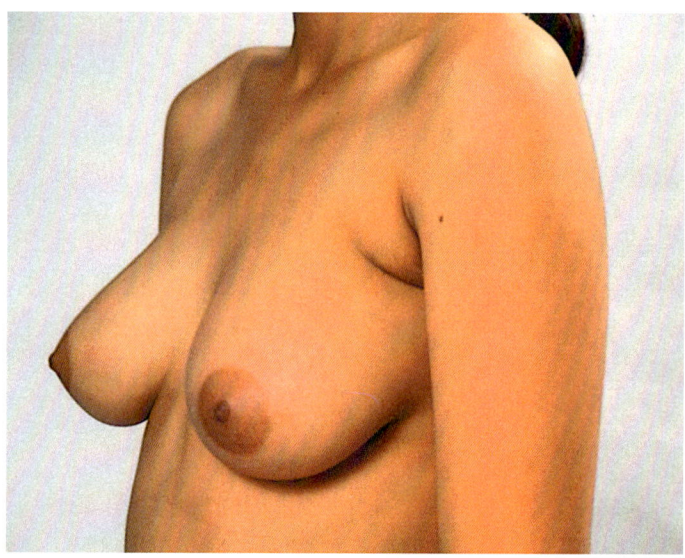
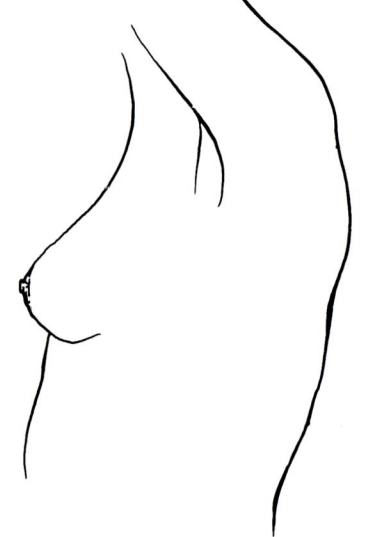
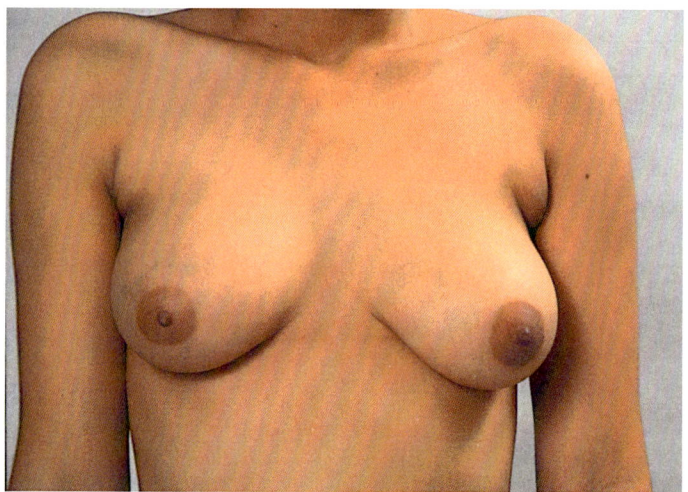

SOURCE: Carlos J. Bourdony, MD, former Director of Pediatric Endocrinology, San Juan City Hospital, San Juan, Puerto Rico.

Staging Pubic Hair Development

Pubic Hair Stage 1
Prepubertal. The vellus over the pubis is no further developed than that over the abdominal wall, ie, no pubic hair.

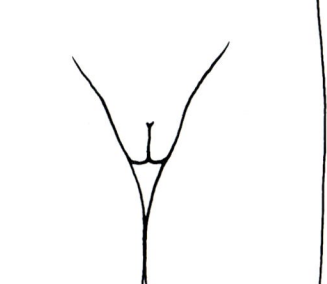
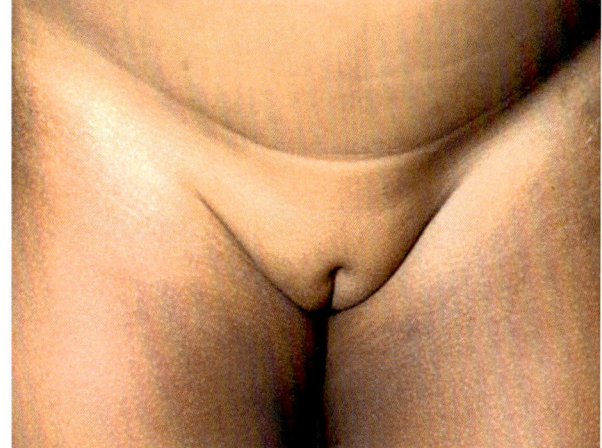

Pubic Hair Stage 2
Sparse growth of slightly pigmented, longer but still downy hair, straight or only slightly curled, appearing chiefly along the labia.

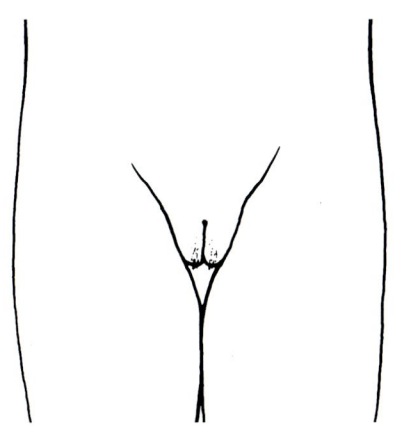
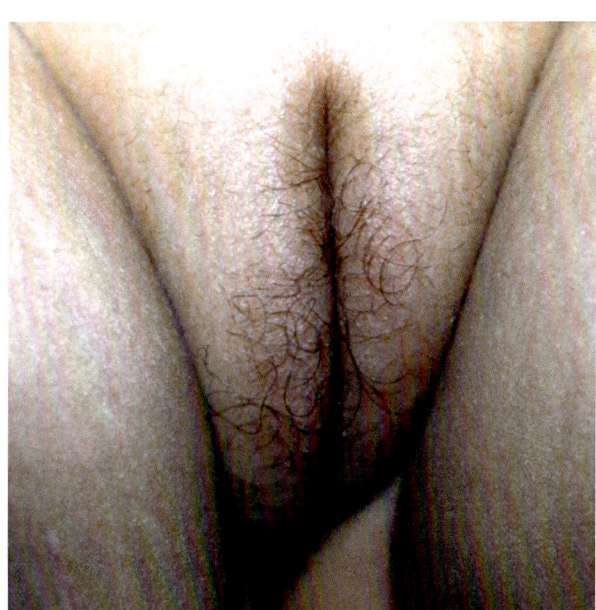

Pubic Hair Stage 3
The hair is considerably darker, coarser, and more curled. The hair spreads sparsely over the mons.

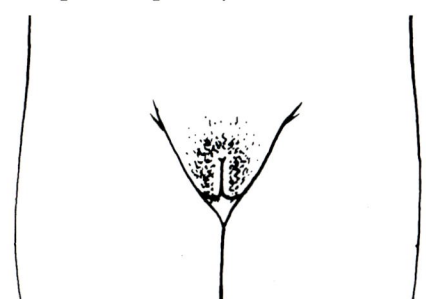
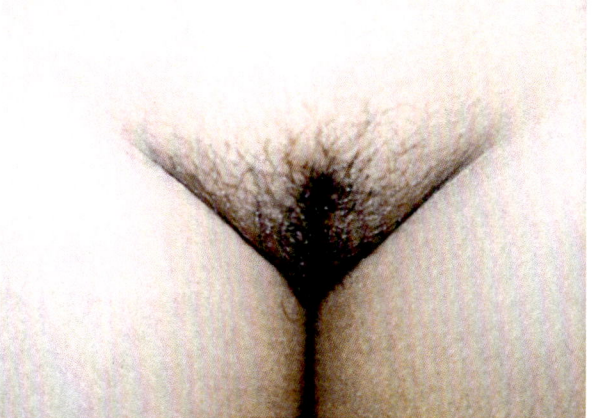

SOURCE: Carlos J. Bourdony, MD, former Director of Pediatric Endocrinology, San Juan City Hospital, San Juan, Puerto Rico.

Pubic Hair Stage 4

The hair now resembles adult type. The area covered is still smaller than that in the adult, but the hair is beginning to spread across the mons. There is no hair spread to the medial thighs.

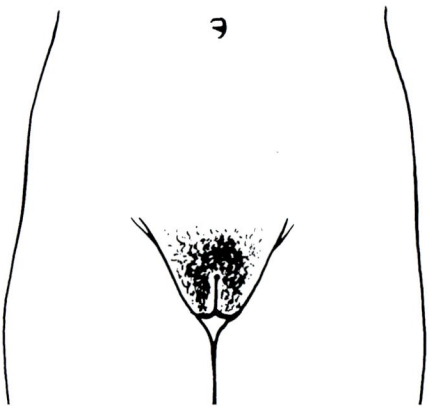
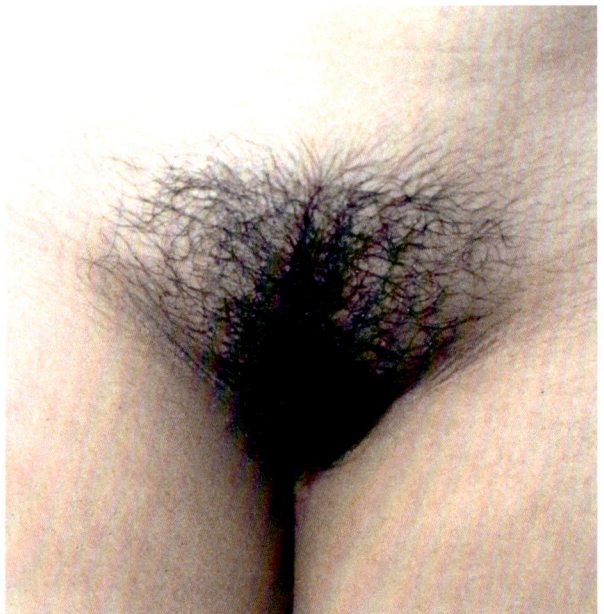

Pubic Hair Stage 5

The hair is adult in type and quantity; darker, coarse, and curled; and distributed in the classic female triangle. Some individuals may have hair spread to the medial thighs.

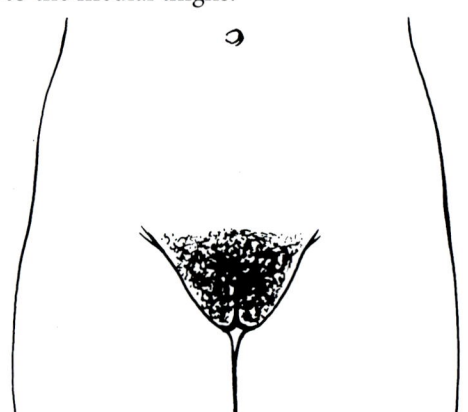
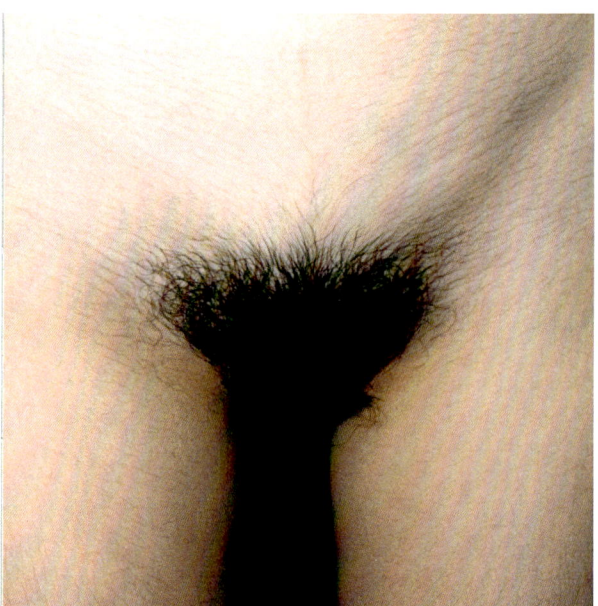

SOURCE: Carlos J. Bourdony, MD, former Director of Pediatric Endocrinology, San Juan City Hospital, San Juan, Puerto Rico.

Staging Axillary Hair Development

There are no widely accepted standards for staging axillary hair development. It is practical to assign 3 stages; Stage 3 is marked by the presence of adult-type hair.

Axillary Hair Stage 1
There is no growth.

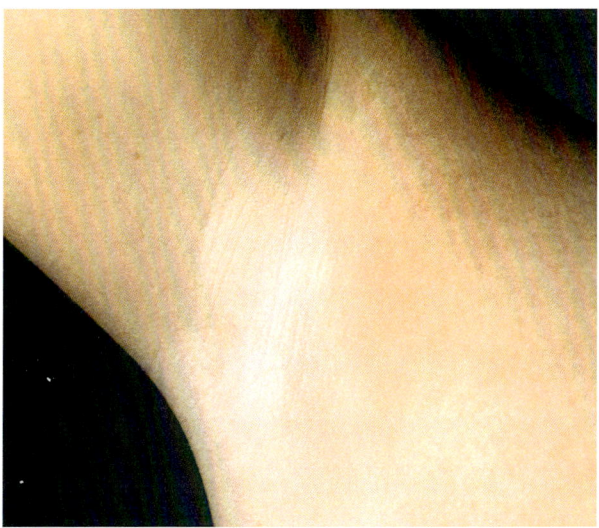

Axillary Hair Stage 2
A sparse amount of straight or slightly curly hair is presented. (In many cultures, young girls may begin shaving axillary hair even at Stage 2, making assessment more difficult.)

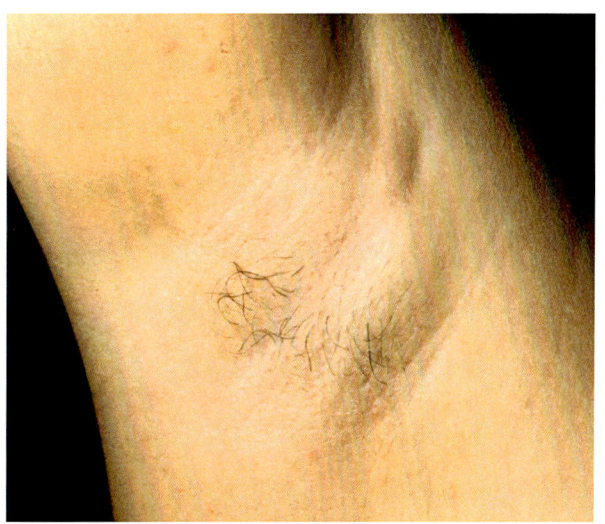

Axillary Hair Stage 3
The hair is adult in type and quality.

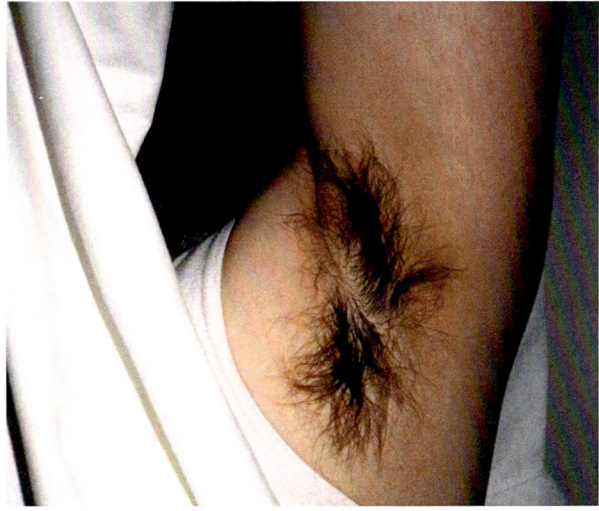

SOURCE: Marcia E. Herman-Giddens, PA, DrPH, adjunct professor in the UNC Gillings School of Global Public Health, Department of Maternal and Child Health, University of North Carolina at Chapel Hill.

Examination Techniques

Breast and Pubic Hair

Tanner staging for the breasts and pubic area is performed as described below. Bras and panties must be removed or temporarily displaced for adequate assessment. There should be good lighting in the room.

The breasts are best examined with the patient sitting. The breast area should be adequately exposed for inspection from the front and side and at an angle. This is best done when auscultation of the heart is being performed. Be sure to note each breast separately.

Since Tanner staging is based on visual inspection only, palpation may not be routinely performed. Certain clinical factors may indicate the need for palpation. For example, in an obese girl, palpation would be needed to differentiate adipose tissue from true breast budding.

If palpation is required, it is best performed by using the second, third, and fourth fingers. The breast should be gently palpated on each side of the areola and then in a circular fashion. Breast tissue is felt as a discrete firm mass under the nipple, 1 cm or more in diameter.

The pubic area is examined with the patient in the supine position. The panties must be removed or sufficiently displaced to allow for clear visualization of the labia majora, where Stage 2 hair usually makes it first appearance. It is essential that lighting be bright, particularly when examining fair-haired girls. Stage 2 is easy to miss in these individuals.

Axillary Hair

Examine both axillae with the patient sitting or lying. Again, good lighting is important.

The Influence of Breast Type

Individuals vary in breast type from small or "flat" to very large. The influence of a girl's basic type on the assessment of the Tanner stage can cause confusion. The figure from the Reynolds and Wines study[18] (p 17) depicts 4 different individuals, each in Stage 5 for breast development.

The Influence of Breast Types on Assessment of Stage of Development

Standards for breast shape. Pair A shows the flat type; B, the hemispherical type; C, the conical type; and D, a distorted type, due to obesity. These 4 girls are all at menarche and are *all* Stage 5.

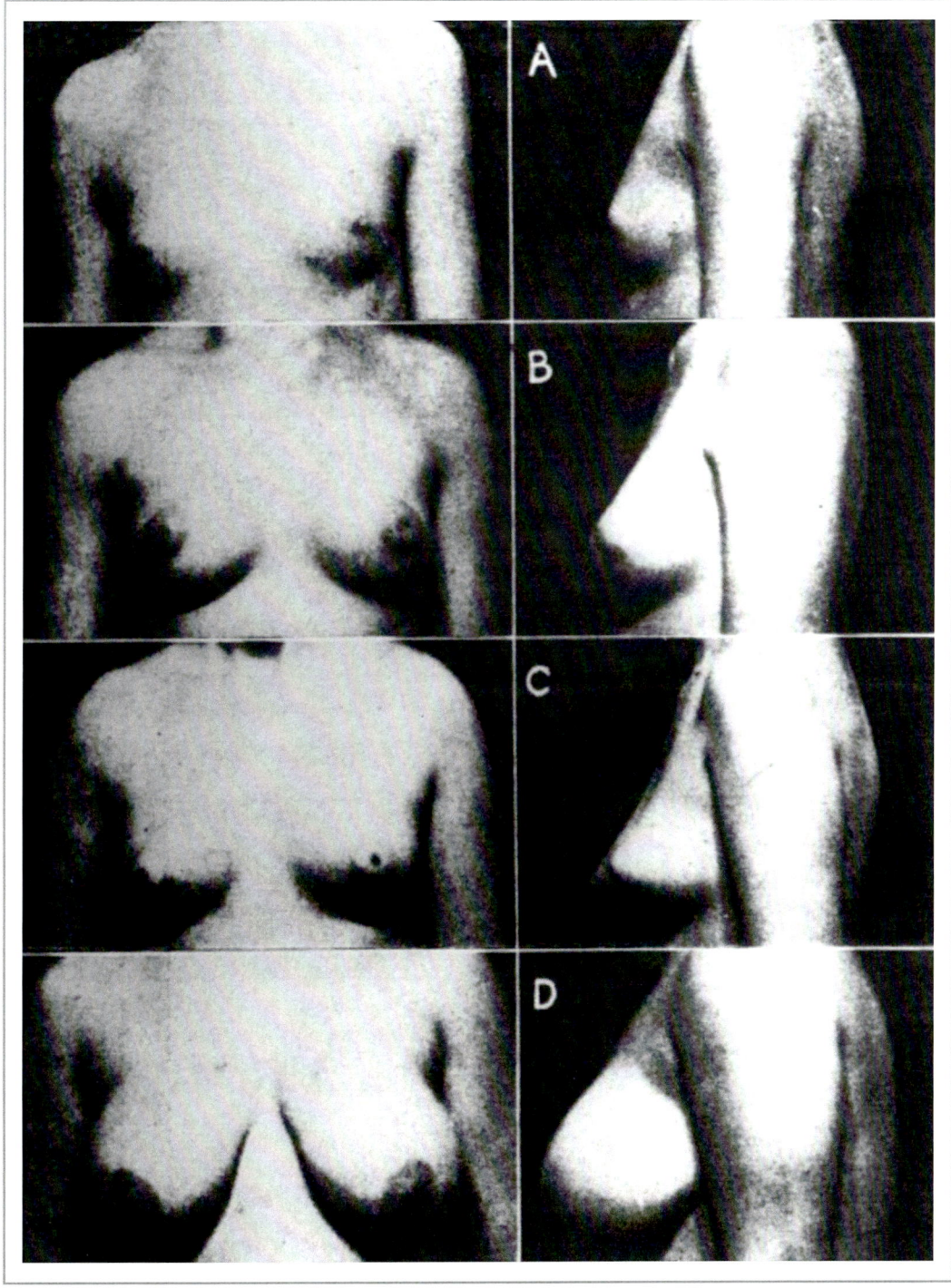

SOURCE: Reprinted by permission from Reynolds EL, Wines JV. Individual differences of physical changes associated with adolescence in girls. *Am J Dis Child*. 1948;75:329–350. Copyright © 1948, American Medical Association. All rights reserved.

Assignment of Stages for Breast and Pubic Hair Development

It is important to be aware that breast and pubic hair development often take place at different rates, especially during the early stages. The breasts themselves may also be at different stages. Therefore, rating of one area should not influence rating of the other. Occasionally, the stages may be quite discrepant.

Breast Anomalies

Occasionally a child may present with unusual breast features. It is helpful to be familiar with these possibilities. Prevalence of these anomalies is unknown.

Anomalies include the following:
- Premature thelarche—Breast development that usually occurs between 6 months and 2 years, distinguished from pubertal development by the presence of a breast bud and absence of other pubertal signs; areolar changes are usually absent.
- Omission of stages of development—Some females appear to stop development at Stage 4, while others appear to go from Stage 3 directly to Stage 5.
- Absence of nipples (athelia).
- Accessory nipples (polythelia).
- Accessory breast tissue (polymastia).
- Asymmetric breast development (anisomastia).
- Absence of the breast (amastia).
- Underdevelopment of the breast (hypoplasia or micromastia).
- Hyperplasia (juvenile and adult types).
- Trunk breast—An unusual malformation constituting marked enlargement of the areola with herniation of the anterior parenchyma into it.
- Inverted nipple.

Pubic Hair Variants

There are few unusual features of pubic hair development.
- Premature pubarche—"Early" development of pubic or axillary hair.
- Premature adrenarche—This term is often used instead of premature pubarche to refer to the "early" appearance of sexual hair. Technically the term refers to early activation of the adrenal cortex, which can be shown by finding higher levels of dehydroepiandrosterone that, in turn, causes the growth of pubic and axillary hair.
- Stage "6"—Some females will develop hair on the lateral thighs or on the area ascending the midline above the mons; occasionally this may be termed Stage 6.

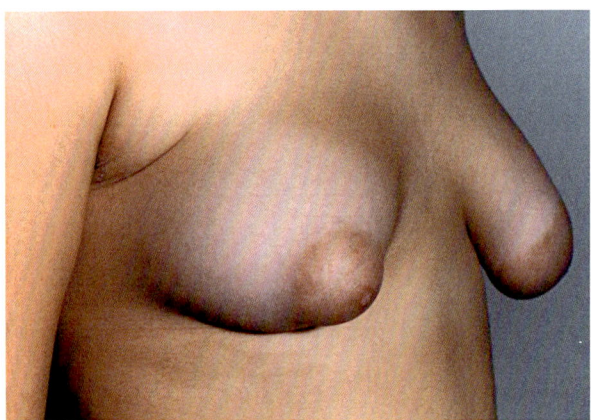

Trunk breast

SOURCE: Carlos J. Bourdony, MD, former Director of Pediatric Endocrinology, San Juan City Hospital, San Juan, Puerto Rico.

Assessment of Sexual Maturity Stages in Boys

Introduction

Observation of the development of genital and pubic hair growth in boys is an essential part of the physical examination. Accurate staging of the physical changes of sexual development provides an important basis for the diagnosis and management of certain clinical problems that may arise as the child grows and matures. In addition, counseling of patients and families regarding the expected timing and sequence of pubertal development depends on accurate physical assessment and understanding of the stages of development. Because gynecomastia is common among and of concern to adolescent boys, assessing breast tissue development may also be important.

The following material demonstrates how to assign the stages of the physical changes of pubertal development using the system described by Marshall and Tanner.[4] We also describe the correct technique for measuring testicular size using orchidometer beads. Since the first (and most objectively measurable) outward sign of puberty in boys is usually testicular growth, it may be difficult to determine by visual inspection alone whether puberty has begun without using other methods for detecting the relatively subtle increase in testicular volume to greater than 3 mL. The prepubertal testis may vary in size from approximately 1 to 2 mL in volume; an increase to 3 or 4 mL is usually accepted as the beginning of pubertal development. While using orchidometer beads is not part of Tanner staging (the latter is based on visual inspection only), the orchidometer provides a fairly accurate and clinically feasible way of assessing the size of the testicles.[19]

Sexual Maturity Ratings

The system of sexual maturity rating presented here is based on the work of Marshall and Tanner.[4,20] This rating system has been widely used for decades in studies around the world. Various schemes for rating the stages of sexual maturity in males appear in medical literature from the 1930s on.[20,21] After the publication of Marshall and Tanner's landmark paper on pubertal changes in boys,[4] the use of the staging methodology defined in that paper became the standard. Genital growth and pubic hair growth are staged separately.

The terms used in describing sexual maturity stages and male anatomy are defined as follows:

Definitions

Areola: the circular, darkly pigmented area of the skin surrounding the nipple

Corpus spongiosum: the spongy body of the penis

Epispadias: the opening of the urethra on the dorsal surface of the penis

Glans penis: the conical expansion of the corpus spongiosum which forms the head of the penis

Gynecomastia: enlargement of the glandular tissue of the breasts in a male (Enlargement of the soft adipose tissue alone in the breasts of a male is called *pseudogynecomastia.*)

Hypospadias: the opening of the urethra on the ventral surface of the glans or on the shaft of the penis proximal to the glans

Linea alba: the fibrous band running vertically along the center of the anterior abdominal wall

Pubes: plural of pubis

Pubis: the region located over the pubic bone, just above the external genitals

Vellus: the fine hair that succeeds the lanugo over most of the body and persists until puberty

Genital Maturity Ratings: The Tanner Photographs

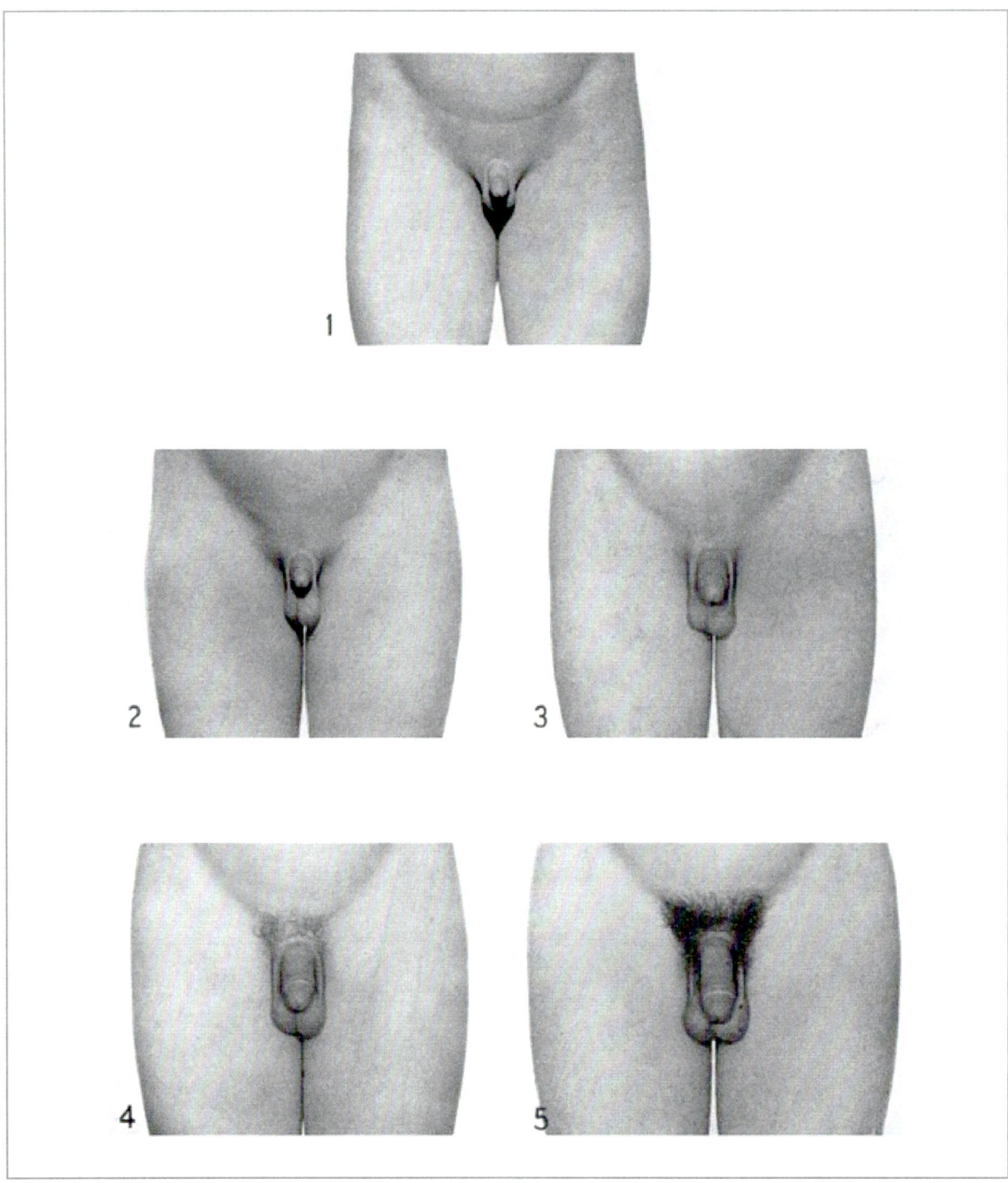

SOURCE: Tanner JM. *Growth at Adolescence*. Oxford, UK: Blackwell Scientific Publications; 1955. Reproduced with permission of Blackwell Publishing Ltd.

NOTE: The quality of the Tanner photos on this page and subsequent pages cannot be improved due to the text source and lack of originals.

Genital Maturity Ratings: The van Wieringen Photographs

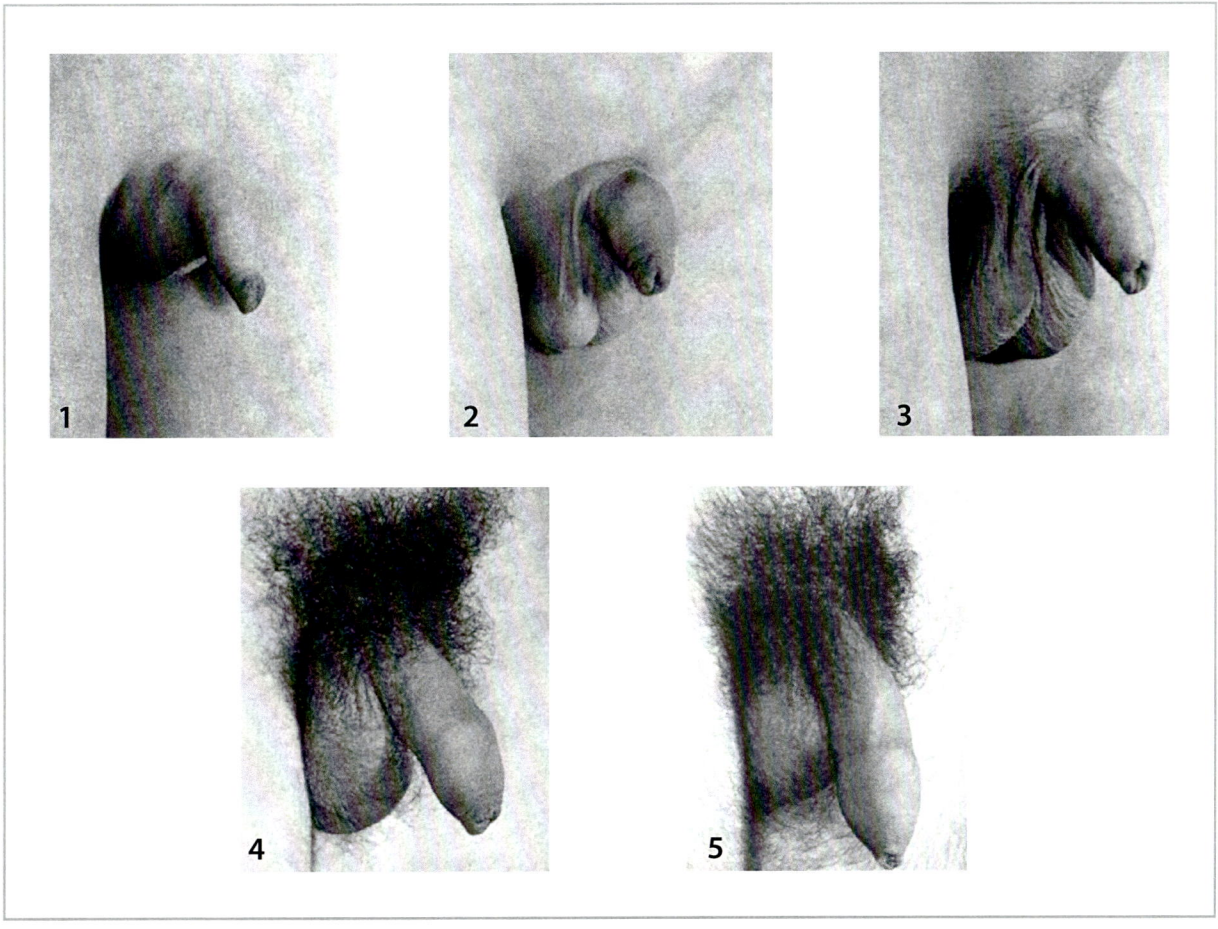

SOURCE: Reprinted by permission from van Wieringen JC, Wafelbakker F, Verbrugge HP, De Haas JH. *Growth Diagrams 1965.* Groningen, The Netherlands: Wolters-Noordhoff; 1971. As included in Yen SSC, Jaffe RB (eds): *Reproductive Endocrinology: Physiology, Pathophysiology and Clinical Management,* 2nd ed. Philadelphia, PA: WB Saunders; 1978. Copyright Elsevier.

Staging Genital Development

The following descriptions, drawings, and photographs should be studied together.

Genital Stage 1

Prepubertal. Penis, testes, and scrotum are about the same size and proportions as in early childhood. Note how the uncircumsized penis may appear larger than it really is. It is important to take this into account when assessing penile growth.

> *Note:* **While studying the text and photographs in this section, focus only on the genitals, *not* the pubic hair. Pubic hair is staged separately as presented in the next section.**

Circumcised

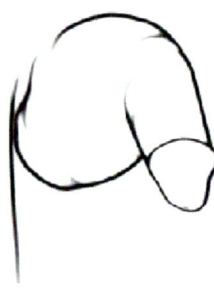
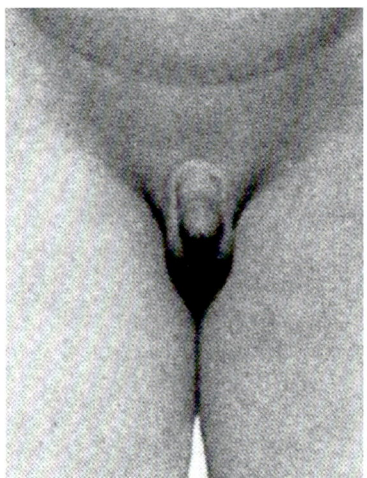

Uncircumcised

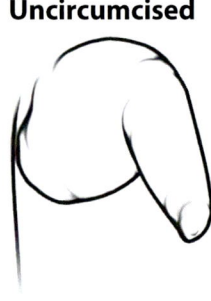
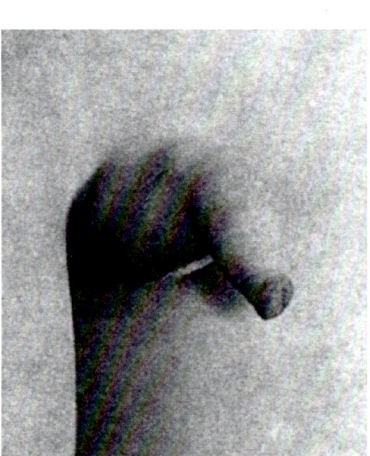

SOURCES:

Circumcised: Tanner JM. *Growth at Adolescence.* Oxford, UK: Blackwell Scientific Publications; 1955. Reproduced with permission of Blackwell Publishing Ltd.

Uncircumcised: Reprinted by permission from van Wieringen JC, Wafelbakker F, Verbrugge HP, De Haas JH. *Growth Diagrams 1965.* Groningen, The Netherlands: Wolters-Noordhoff; 1971. As included in Yen SSC, Jaffe RB (eds): *Reproductive Endocrinology: Physiology, Pathophysiology and Clinical Management,* 2nd ed. Philadelphia, PA: WB Saunders; 1978. Copyright Elsevier.

Genital Stage 2

Only the testes and scrotum have begun to enlarge from the early childhood size. The penis is still prepubertal in appearance. The texture of the scrotal skin is beginning to become thinner and the skin appears redder due to increased vascularization.

Circumcised   **Uncircumcised**

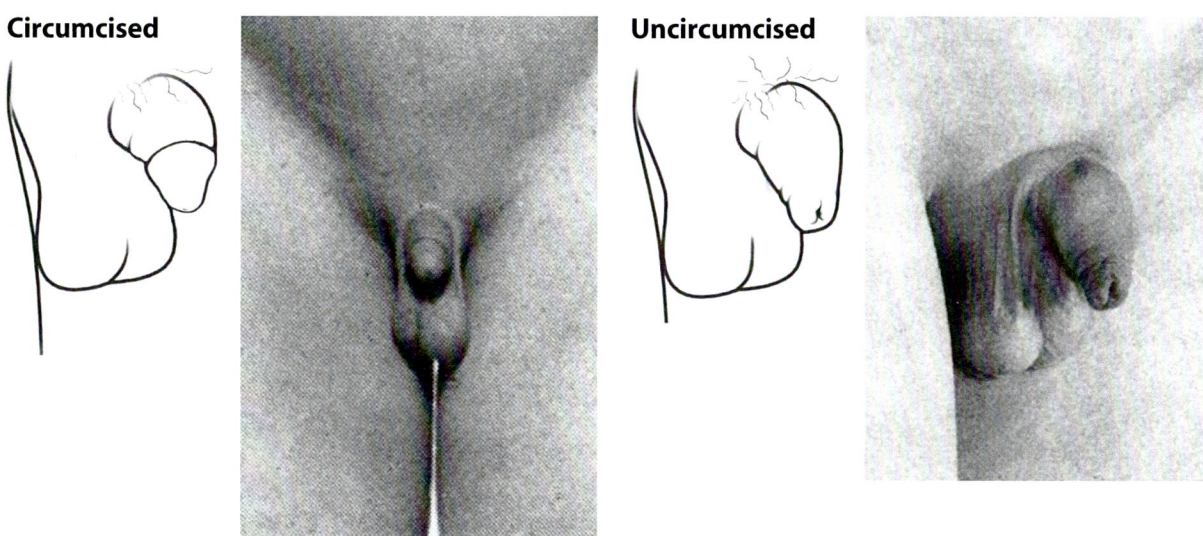

Genital Stage 3

There is further growth of the testes and scrotum. The penis is also beginning to grow, mainly in length with some increase in breadth. It can be difficult to distinguish between stages 2 and 3.

Circumcised   **Uncircumcised**

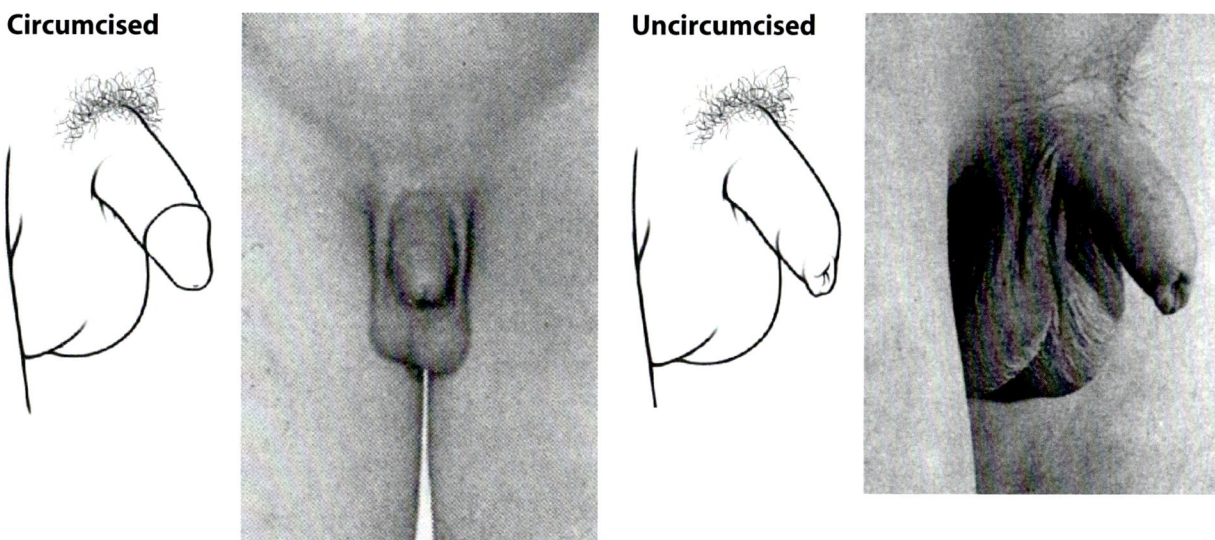

SOURCES:
Circumcised: Tanner JM. *Growth at Adolescence.* Oxford, UK: Blackwell Scientific Publications; 1955. Reproduced with permission of Blackwell Publishing Ltd.

Uncircumcised: Reprinted by permission from van Wieringen JC, Wafelbakker F, Verbrugge HP, De Haas JH. *Growth Diagrams 1965.* Groningen, The Netherlands: Wolters-Noordhoff; 1971. As included in Yen SSC, Jaffe RB (eds): *Reproductive Endocrinology: Physiology, Pathophysiology and Clinical Management,* 2nd ed. Philadelphia, PA: WB Saunders; 1978. Copyright Elsevier.

Genital Stage 4

The penis enlarges further in length and breadth and the glans becomes more prominent. The testes and scrotum are larger. There is further darkening of the scrotal skin.

> *Note:* **The photo and the drawing on the right demonstrate an example of a discrepancy between genital and pubic hair stages. The genitals are Stage 4, and the pubic hair is Stage 5.**

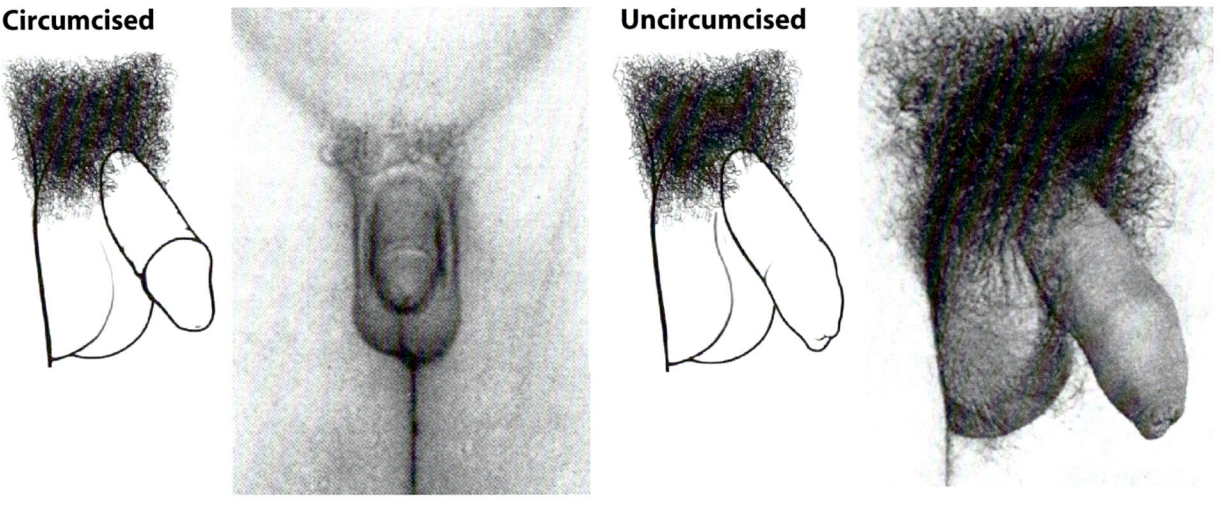

Genital Stage 5

The penis, testes, and scrotum are adult in size and shape.

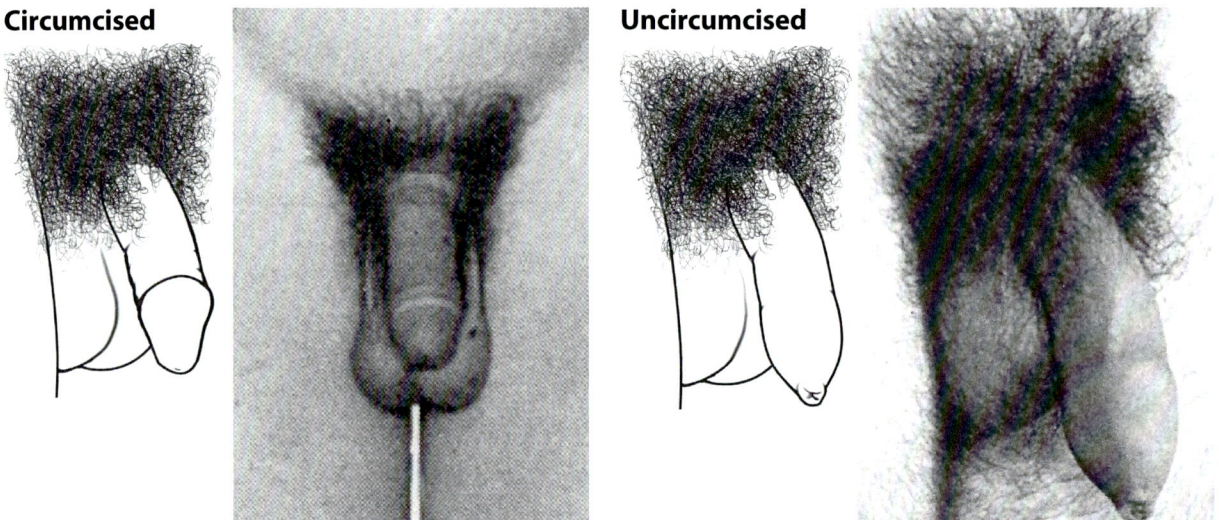

SOURCES:
Circumcised: Tanner JM. *Growth at Adolescence.* Oxford, UK: Blackwell Scientific Publications; 1955. Reproduced with permission of Blackwell Publishing Ltd.

Uncircumcised: Reprinted by permission from van Wieringen JC, Wafelbakker F, Verbrugge HP, De Haas JH. *Growth Diagrams 1965.* Groningen, The Netherlands: Wolters-Noordhoff; 1971. As included in Yen SSC, Jaffe RB (eds): *Reproductive Endocrinology: Physiology, Pathophysiology and Clinical Management,* 2nd ed. Philadelphia, PA: WB Saunders; 1978. Copyright Elsevier.

Staging Pubic Hair Growth

Pubic Hair Stage 1

Prepubertal. The vellus over the pubis is similar to that on the abdomen. This hair has not yet developed the characteristics of pubic hair.

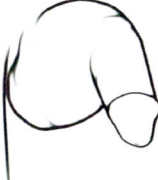
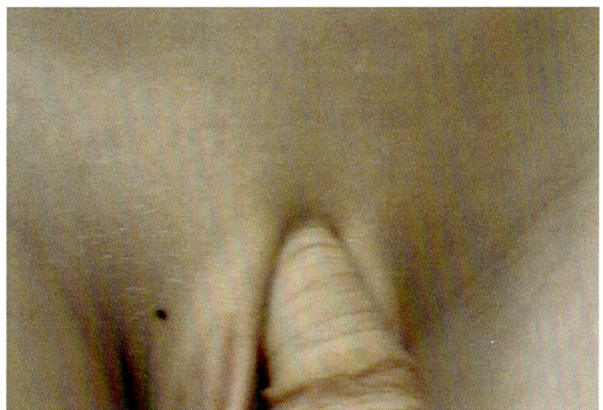

SOURCE: Reprinted by permission from John S. Fuqua, MD, associate professor of clinical pediatrics, Section of Pediatric Endocrinology and Diabetology, Department of Pediatrics, Indiana University School of Medicine and Riley Hospital for Children, Indianapolis.

Pubic Hair Stage 2

There is sparse growth of long, slightly pigmented downy hair, straight or only slightly curled, mainly at the base of the penis.

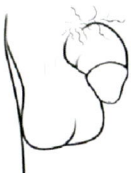
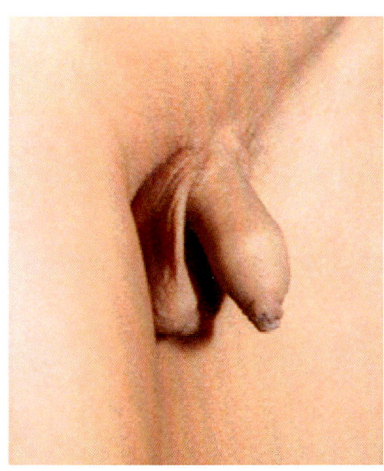

SOURCE: Carlos J. Bourdony, MD, former Director of Pediatric Endocrinology, San Juan City Hospital, San Juan, Puerto Rico.

Pubic Hair Stage 3

The hair is considerably darker, coarser, and more curled. It is spread sparsely over the pubis.

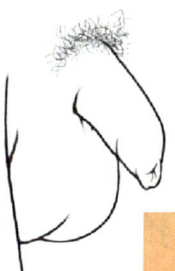
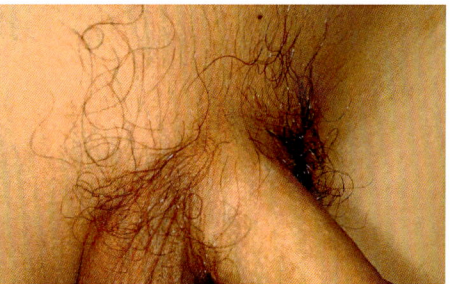

SOURCE: Marsha L. Davenport, MD, professor of pediatrics, Division of Pediatric Endocrinology, Department of Pediatrics, and Medical Illustrations, University of North Carolina School of Medicine, Chapel Hill.

Pubic Hair Stage 4

The hair is adult in type but the area over which it is present is smaller than in most adults. It has not yet spread to the medial thighs or along the linea alba.

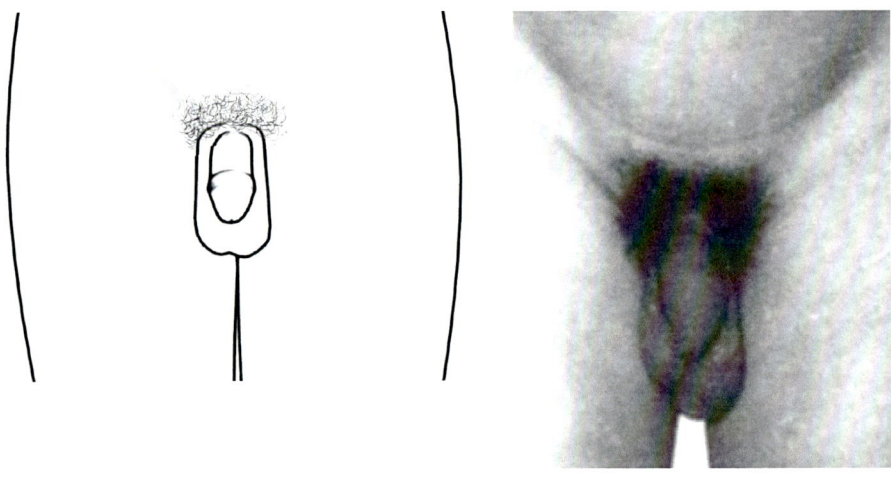

Pubic Hair Stage 5

The hair is adult in quality and quantity and has the classical triangular distribution. It may spread to the medial surface of the thighs. It has not spread up the linea alba.*

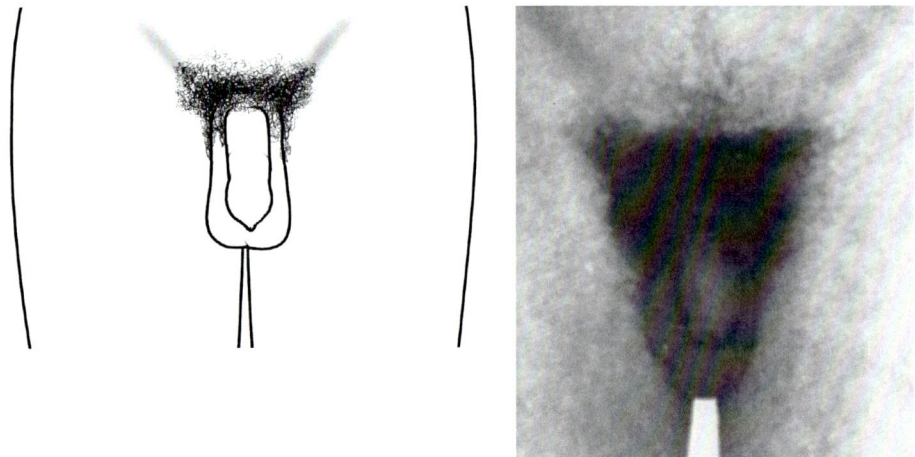

SOURCE: Tanner JM. *Growth at Adolescence*. Oxford, UK: Blackwell Scientific Publications; 1955. Reproduced with permission of Blackwell Publishing Ltd.

NOTE: The quality of the Tanner photos on this page and subsequent pages cannot be improved due to the text source and lack of originals.

---

*In about 80% of males, the pubic hair spreads up the linea alba some time after Stage 5 has been reached. This is sometimes referred to as Stage 6. The final adult pubic hair pattern may not be reached until the mid-20s.[4]

Examples of Subtleties of Staging

This boy was assessed as Tanner Stage 1 for pubic hair and genitalia by his pediatric endocrinologist. There is no visible pubic hair, so an assignment of pubic hair Stage 1 is clear. However, due to the lack of scale and some thinness of the scrotal skin, from the photograph alone it could be argued that the genitalia are Stage 1 or Stage 2.

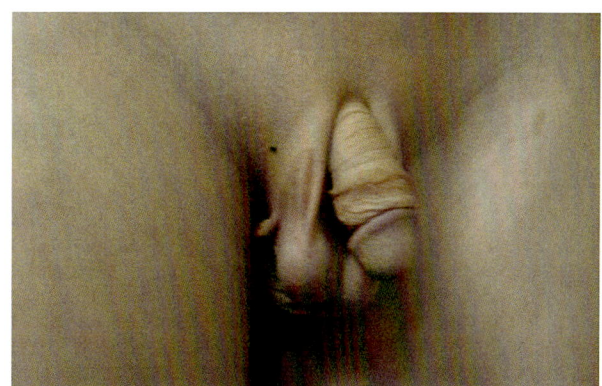

This boy is pubic hair Stage 1 and genitalia Stage 2. Note the partial erection, which is not an uncommon occurrence during examinations as discussed in "Examination Techniques" on page 32. The examiner must be careful not to be falsely influenced in assigning the genital stage when this occurs. In this photograph, testicular size is easier to assess because more of the subject is shown, providing some sense of proportion.

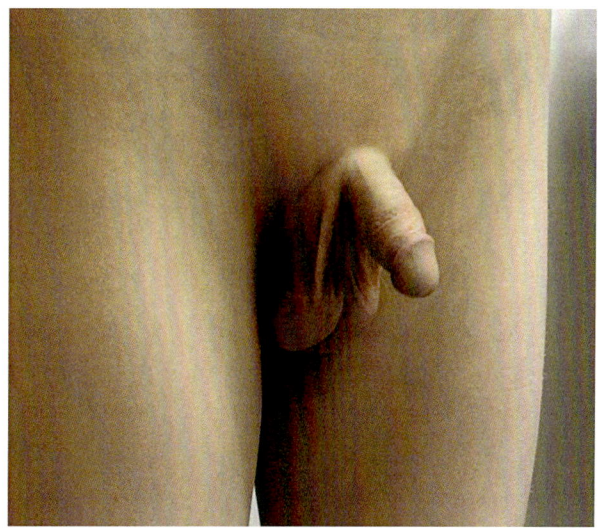

This photograph shows pubic hair Stage 2 and genitalia Stage 3 as determined from the clinical examination. In the photograph the few wisps of pubic hair that are visible make the child's pubic hair development clearly Stage 2. The subject has not reached Stage 4 with its darker scrotal skin and near mature penile and testicular size. The penis appears to be too broad and long for Stage 2 genitalia, although without a scale some might rate this as Stage 2.

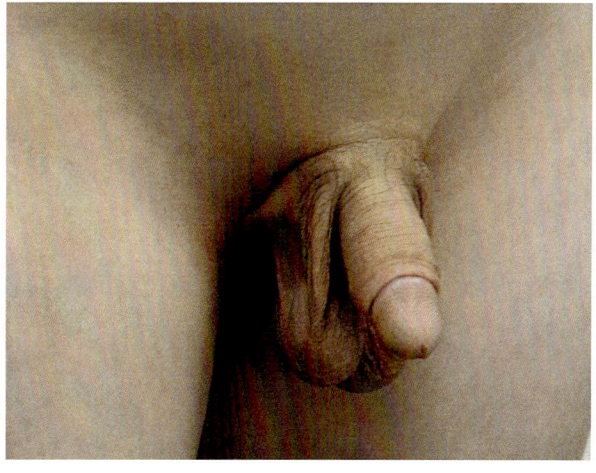

SOURCE: John S. Fuqua, MD, associate professor of clinical pediatrics, Section of Pediatric Endocrinology and Diabetology, Department of Pediatrics, Indiana University School of Medicine and Riley Hospital for Children, Indianapolis.

This boy was assessed as pubic hair Stage 4 and genitalia Stage 3 by his pediatric endocrinologist. Some examiners might consider the pubic hair between a Stage 3 and 4, and grade it as Stage 3-4 or 3+. In pubertal studies where gradations cannot be used, the lower number is usually used. In "real life," because the growth of pubic hair and genitalia is a continuum, many children will, of course, be between the classic stages as described by Marshall and Tanner.[4]

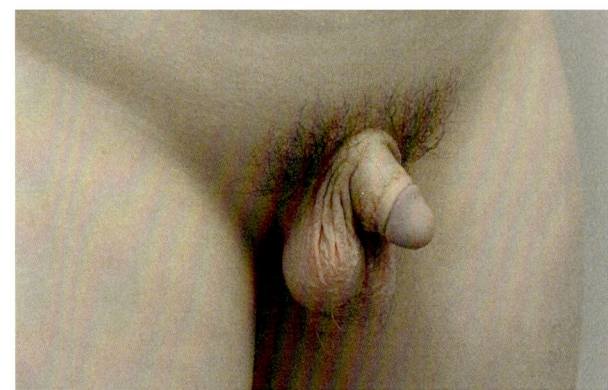

This boy was assessed as Tanner Stage 3 pubic hair. Though there is more than the requisite amount of hair for Stage 3, it has not started to spread up the pubis.

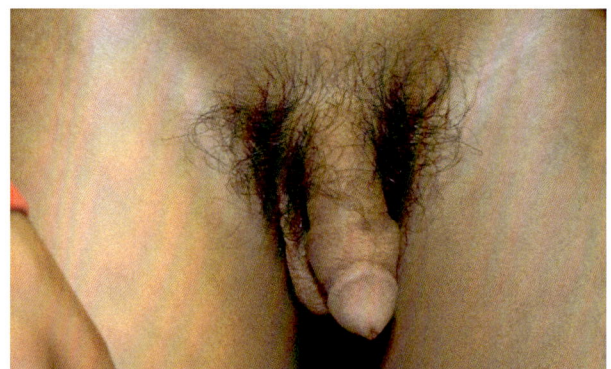

Pubic hair Stage 5 is clearly shown in this photograph. This subject was considered to be genitalia Stage 4 by his endocrinologist; however, an assessment made from the photograph could be Stage 3.

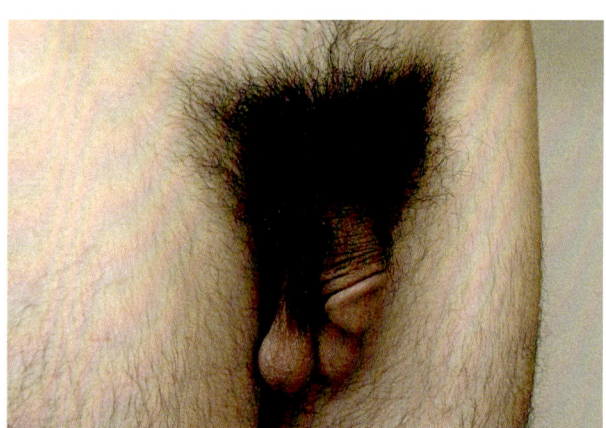

This boy was assessed as Stage 5. The photograph shows an example of a morbidly obese boy for whom it is necessary to lift the panniculus for complete assessment of the genitalia and pubic hair.

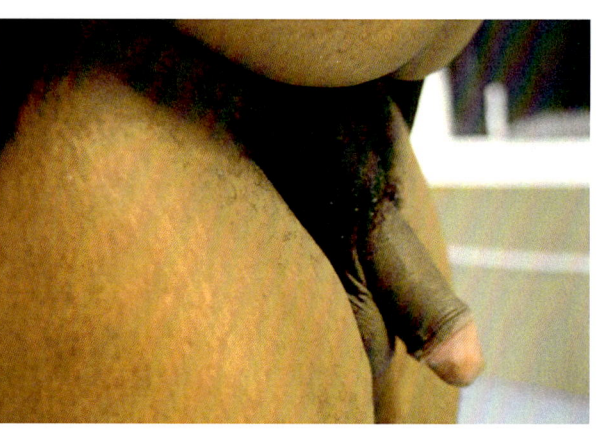

SOURCES: First and third images: John S. Fuqua, MD, associate professor of clinical pediatrics, Section of Pediatric Endocrinology and Diabetology, Department of Pediatrics, Indiana University School of Medicine and Riley Hospital for Children, Indianapolis.

Second and fourth images: Marsha L. Davenport, MD, and Anita Azam, MD, Division of Pediatric Endocrinology, University of North Carolina, and Mr Earl Nichols, Chapel Hill, NC.

Staging Axillary Hair Development

There are no widely accepted standards for staging axillary hair development. It is practical to assign 3 stages; Stage 3 is marked by the presence of adult-type hair.

Axillary Hair Stage 1
There is no growth.

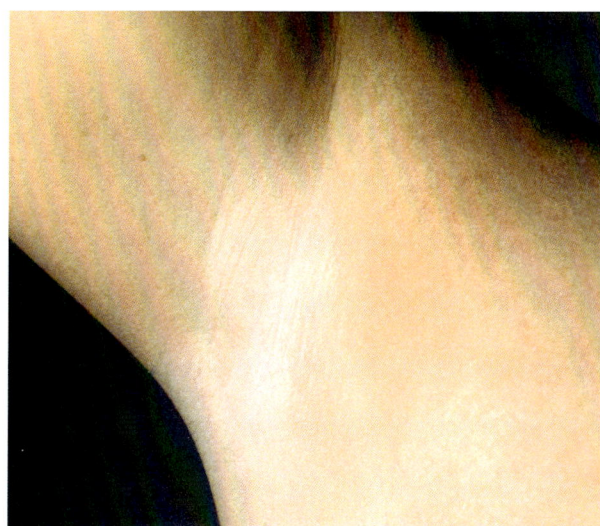

Axillary Hair Stage 2
A sparse amount of straight or slightly curly hair is presented.

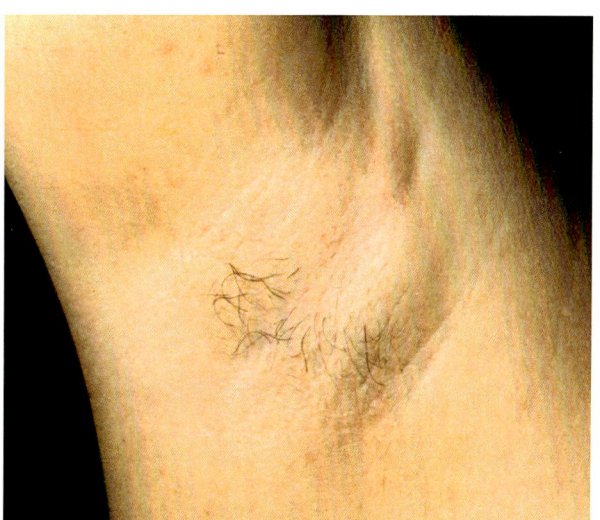

Axillary Hair Stage 3
The hair is adult in type and quality.

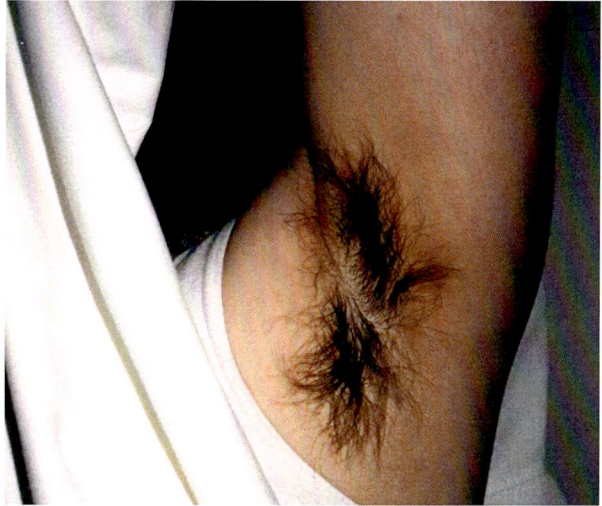

SOURCE: Marcia E. Herman-Giddens, PA, DrPH, adjunct professor in the UNC Gillings School of Global Public Health, Department of Maternal and Child Health, University of North Carolina at Chapel Hill.

Examination Techniques

Staging of the physical changes of pubertal maturation in boys is somewhat more difficult than the staging of girls because it is primarily based on relatively subjective assessments of changes in genital size and scrotal skin characteristics rather than the more readily distinguishable changes in breast contour seen in girls. If the boy's physical development is not followed longitudinally, staging may be difficult when done at a one-point-in-time examination, given that at any stage of development, there is at least a twofold range in testicular size in normal males of all ages. The range of normal for penile size varies as well. Another challenge is that genital development and pubic hair growth must be staged separately; therefore, *it is important that the examiner not let his or her assessment of one feature influence the assessment of the other.*

Anatomy: A Brief Review

Several features of male anatomy are important to understand in learning to assess genital maturation.

Scrotum
This fibromuscular sac contains a partial median septum that separates the pockets that contain each testis.

Testicular Size
Normal testicular volume ranges from 0.6 to 1.3 mL in early childhood.[22] At sexual maturity testicular size ranges from about 11 to 22 mL in volume. On average, the ovoid adult testis is approximately 4 to 5 cm long and 2 to 3 cm wide. A volume of 25 mL is considered the upper limit of normal. The left testis usually hangs lower than the right, and the right testis is often slightly larger. The testes are covered by several layers of tissue. The epididymis is a soft comma-shaped structure that houses the spermatozoa. Its head sits along the top of the testis while the body and tail extend along the side of the testis to where it connects to the vas deferens. These structures add to the perceived size of the testis when visually inspected or palpated.

Penile Size
Stretched penile length ranges from about 3 to 7 cm in early childhood. The mature stretched penile length ranges from about 11 to 15 cm.[22] Reynolds and Wines found that some boys have a regression in penile size after reaching Stage 5 in maturity.[21] The true penile size may be obscured in the overweight or obese boy due to the prominence of the perineal fat pad.

Anomalies and Conditions That May Be Encountered When Assessing Pubertal Maturation in Males

Penis/Scrotum
Hypospadias: A congenital condition in which the urethral opening is located on the inferior (ventral) surface of the glans or shaft of the penis.

Chordee: Commonly associated with hypospadias, is the ventral curvature of the penis due to the presence of tough fibrous bands.

Epispadias: A congenital condition in which the urethral opening is located on the dorsal surface of the penis. This is much less common that hypospadias.

Micropenis: A stretched penile length of less than 2 cm at birth (defined as <-2.5 SD for age).

Adherent penis: Also known as webbing, results from the attachment of the scrotum to the ventral surface of the penile shaft. The penis may be small or appear to be small.

Position: In some adolescents the penis does not hang vertically, but may hang markedly to the left or right.

Testis

Size and position: The left testis is usually slightly smaller and hangs lower than the right.

Cryptorchidism: Undescended testis. The condition may be unilateral or bilateral. This must be distinguished from a retractile testis (see below). An undescended testis may reside anywhere along the developmental course of testicular descent, from the abdominal cavity to the upper scrotum. An undescended testis is often smaller than normal due to dysgenesis (abnormal development of the testis). An ectopic testis is a testis that is not located along the normal course of testicular descent, such as in the femoral area.

Polyorchidism: The presence of more than one testis on one or both sides of the scrotum. Triorchidism is the most common variant, but up to 5 testes have been reported.

Retractile testis: A testis that on examination is in a position outside the scrotum (or in the upper part of the scrotum) but that can be manually manipulated into the normal position in the scrotal sac. This is thought to be due to an exaggerated cremasteric reflex. These testes are more likely to retract when a cremasteric reflex is triggered by exposure to cold environmental temperatures, anxiety, or other factors. After puberty, a formerly retractile testis will continuously reside in a normal position in the scrotal sac.

Varicocele: The "bag of worms" scrotal mass caused by dilation of the spermatic vein due to the incompetence of valves in the vein. This usually presents as a painless bluish mass.

Hydrocele: A non-tender fluid-filled mass occupying the space within the tunica vaginalis or the processus vaginalis of the spermatic cord. The mass transilluminates.

Atrophy: A testis may atrophy as a result of testicular torsion or other insult or injury.

Hernias may present as scrotal masses. Very rarely, a prepubertal boy will present with a testicular mass from acute lymphobastic leukemia or paratesticular rhabdomyosarcoma. A normal to small penis and small firm testes may indicate Klinefelter syndrome.

Gynecomastia

The diameter of the areola enlarges during puberty and is a normal finding. Up to one third of adolescent males will have a transitory enlargement of the breasts marked by the presence of firm subareolar glandular tissue. This generally appears around the midpoint of pubertal development. Regression usually occurs within a year or so. Asymmetry may be present. The presence of glandular breast tissue must be distinguished from breast enlargement solely due to excess adipose tissue (pseudogynecomastia) by palpation. Although nearly all cases of gynecomastia in adolescents are physiologic, transient, and only of cosmetic concern, in a few cases true or apparent gynecomastia may be due to endocrine disorders, drugs (eg, phenothiazines, marijuana) or tumors. All cases of gynecomastia in prepubertal boys should be considered pathologic, requiring further evaluation.

Examination of Breasts, Genitalia, and Pubic and Axillary Hair

General

Examination of the breasts for gynecomastia takes place while the patient is supine or sitting. Tanner staging of the genitalia and pubic hair takes place at the completion of the physical examination. The patient must have pants removed and underwear at least pulled down to the knees. The room and the examiner's hands should be warm and the lighting must be bright.

Effects of Obesity

The breast and genital examination will be more difficult in the overweight or obese boy. The perineal fat pad may obscure true penile size and adipose tissue can be difficult to distinguish from true breast tissue without careful palpation. Therefore, extra care is required in the examination of the overweight boy.

Gynecomastia

Examine the breast with the patient supine or sitting. To palpate for breast tissue, use the second, third, and fourth fingers to gently palpate both sides of the areola, feeling for the presence of a firm disc of glandular breast tissue. It may also be helpful to lightly grasp the tissue beneath the areola from the sides between the thumb and fingers to assess diameter and help distinguish firm glandular tissue from softer adipose tissue. The tissue may be tender, especially when the breast tissue has been undergoing rapid enlargement.

Pubic Hair

The pubic area may be examined with the patient supine or when he is standing for the genital examination. It is essential to have good lighting.

Genitalia

The genitalia are best inspected at the end of the physical examination. Have the patient stand. In a boy who is not cold or tense, the scrotum is usually loose and the testes can be easily inspected and palpated. Inspect for signs of scrotal skin changes and scrotal and penile enlarging prior to assessing the size of the testes with the orchidometer (described in "Using the Orchidometer"). It is best to palpate the testes soon after pulling down the boy's underwear, since retraction of the testes that may occur with exposure to the air may make it difficult to examine them properly. Retractile testes may not be felt in the scrotum but can usually be manipulated into the scrotal sac. The retraction results from an exaggerated cremasteric reflex stimulated by anxiety or a cold environment and is common in prepubertal boys. If it is difficult to manipulate the testis into the sac, have the boy sit on a chair with his knees pulled up and feet on the edge of the seat for a few minutes. Be sure the room and examiner's hands are warm. It is also common for boys (pubertal and prepubertal) to experience penile erection when the genitalia are being examined, regardless of the gender of the examiner. If this occurs and the boy appears embarrassed or upset, he should be reassured that this is normal and of no concern.

Axillary Hair

Examine both axillae with the patient sitting or supine.

Assignment of Stages for Genital and Pubic Hair Development

It is important to be aware that genital and pubic hair development may take place at different rates. Therefore, rating of one area should not influence rating of the other. In general, genital growth begins before the appearance of pubic hair in boys. Be aware that erections are common in young boys during examination, so it is important to take into account how this influences penile size when assessing sexual maturity stages for the genitalia.

Observation of Voice Change, Facial Hair, and Acne

Voice Change

Voice change is gradual and is related to the enlargement of the larynx that occurs due to testosterone stimulation. Note whether the voice is intermittently "cracking" or consistently deeper. Maximum change usually occurs between genital stages 3 and 4; however, the correlation is somewhat weak.[23]

Facial Hair

Facial hair usually begins to grow at about the same time as axillary hair, about 2 years after the onset of pubic hair growth. Observe the upper lip where the first hair usually appears, then the upper cheeks and the midline just below the lower lip. Hair along the sides of the face and lower chin occurs late in puberty.

Acne

Acne may occur on the face, chest, and back; therefore, observe these areas while performing the rest of the physical examination. More than 90% of adolescent males in Western cultures have some degree of acne. There are many grading systems but, for general purposes, classification from "no acne present" to "severe" without distinguishing the types of pustules suffices. Smithard et al[24] adapted the following method from the Leeds Classification System[25]:

No acne present: <7 easily visible lesions
Mild: 7–20 lesions
Moderate to severe: >20 lesions

Prominent follicles or small milia are not counted.

Using the Orchidometer

The orchidometer is a set of beads first designed and described by Prader in 1966[19] that correspond to testicular volumes of 1 through 25 mL. Other methods of measurement include rulers, calipers, and ultrasound, which is the most accurate. Comparing a testicle held in one hand to a bead in the other is reasonably accurate, less time consuming, and probably more psychologically acceptable than the other methods.

For purposes of establishing whether a boy has begun puberty as indicated by testicular volume, a modified orchidometer can be used and may be more acceptable to the patient.

The normal range of testicular size at each stage varies among individuals at least twofold—0.6 to 1.3 mL in early childhood, to 11 to 22 mL in adulthood. Therefore, assessing whether a particular boy has begun the testicular enlargement of puberty using only visual inspection is too inaccurate. The takeoff point for pubertal testicular growth is generally agreed to be when the testes are >3 mL in volume although a few studies have used ≥3 mL.[26,27]

Because testicular volume does not directly correspond to any specific Tanner stage, the visual assessment of the Tanner stage and testicular volume measurement are desirable to more accurately assess pubertal development, particularly its onset.

Technique

Show the patient the beads and explain the procedure. Let him examine the beads if he wishes. Explain that each testicle will be compared to several beads to see which one it matches. Do not talk about measuring size. When ready to use the orchidometer, have the patient stand. The examiner sits on a chair in front of the patient.

Assess the Tanner stage of the genitalia after the patient is standing. This is also a good time to stage the pubic hair growth if it has not been done previously.

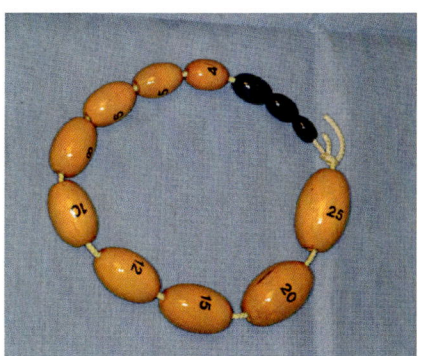

Complete orchidometer

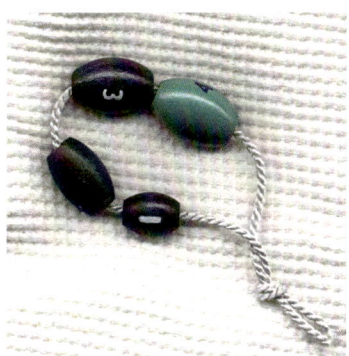

Modified orchidometer

SOURCE: Marcia E. Herman-Giddens, PA, DrPH, adjunct professor in the UNC Gillings School of Global Public Health, Department of Maternal and Child Health, University of North Carolina at Chapel Hill.

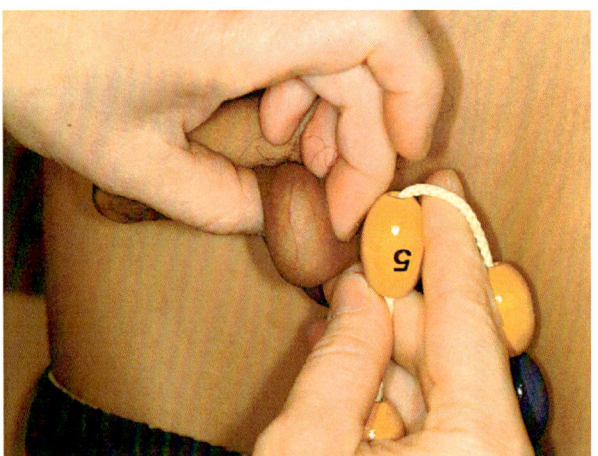

Gently grasp the testicle between the thumb and third finger while holding the orchidometer beads in the opposite hand. Manipulate the testis to expose it for comparison as shown.

Opposing the fingertips just behind the testis should result in gentle stretching of the scrotal skin over the anterior surface of the testis, permitting more accurate measurement.

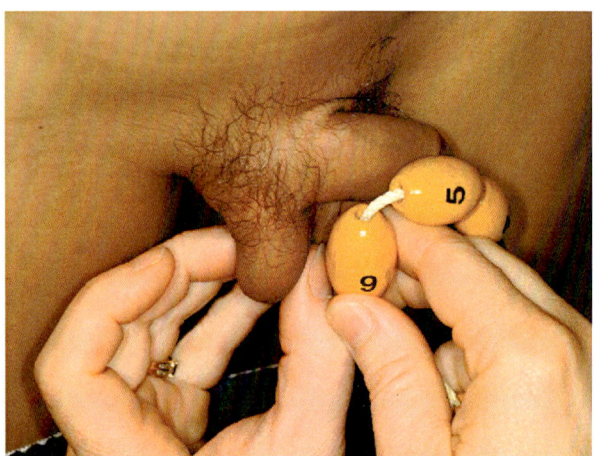

Start with a bead that is likely to be smaller than the testicle.

While maintaining the grasp, maneuver to a bead with a higher number to assess for a better match.

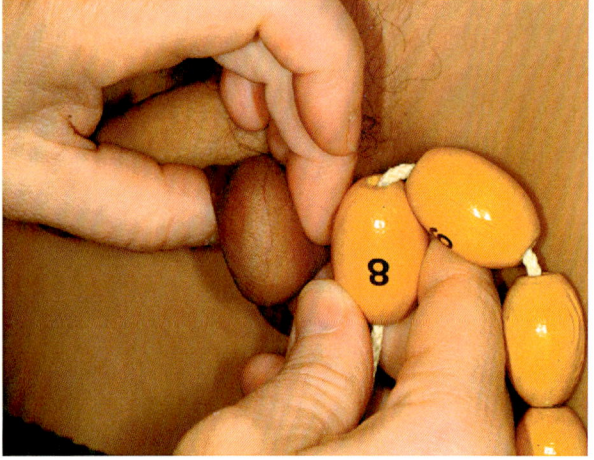

Further check by comparing with the next larger bead. Record as appropriate.

Repeat for the opposite testis. Record right and left separately.

SOURCE: Marsha L. Davenport, MD, professor of pediatrics, Division of Pediatric Endocrinology, Department of Pediatrics, and Medical Illustrations, University of North Carolina School of Medicine, Chapel Hill.

References

1. Herman-Giddens ME, Bourdony CJ. *Assessment of Sexual Maturity Stages in Girls.* Elk Grove Village, IL: Pediatric Research in Office Settings, American Academy of Pediatrics; 1995
2. Herman-Giddens ME, Bourdony CJ. *Assessment of Sexual Maturity Stages in Boys.* Elk Grove Village, IL: Pediatric Research in Office Settings, American Academy of Pediatrics; 2005
3. Marshall WA, Tanner JM. Variations in pattern of pubertal changes in girls. *Arch Dis Child.* 1969;44:291–303
4. Marshall WA, Tanner JM. Variations in the pattern of pubertal changes in boys. *Arch Dis Child.* 1970;45:13–23
5. Tanner JM. *Growth at Adolescence.* Oxford, United Kingdom: Blackwell Scientific Publications; 1955
6. van Wieringen JC, Wafelbakker F, Verbrugge HP, De Haas JH. *Growth Diagrams 1965.* Groningen, The Netherlands: Wolters-Noordhoff; 1971. As included in Yen SSC, Jaffe RB, eds. *Reproductive Endocrinology: Physiology, Pathophysiology and Clinical Management.* 2nd ed. Philadelphia, PA: WB Saunders; 1978
7. Tanner JM. Physical growth and development. In: Forfar JO, Arneil GC, eds. *Textbook of Pediatrics.* Vol 1. 3rd ed. Edinburgh, Scotland: Churchill Livingstone; 1984:292–298
8. Villarreal SF, Martorell R, Mendoza F. Sexual maturation of Mexican-American adolescents. *Am J Hum Biol.* 1989;1:87–95
9. Herman-Giddens ME, MacMillan JP. Prevalence of secondary sexual characteristics in a population of North Carolina girls ages 3 to 10. *Adolesc Pediatr Gynecol.* 1991;4:21–26
10. Herman-Giddens ME, Slora EJ, Wasserman RC, et al. Secondary sexual characteristics and menses in young girls seen in office practice: a study from the Pediatric Research in Office Settings network. *Pediatrics.* 1997;99:505–512
11. Billewicz WZ, Fellowes HM, Thomson AM. Pubertal changes in boys and girls in Newcastle upon Tyne. *Ann Hum Biol.* 1981;8:211–219
12. Belmaker E. Sexual maturation of Jerusalem schoolgirls and its association with socio-economic factors and ethnic group. *Ann Hum Biol.* 1982;9:321–328
13. Dacou-Voutetakis C, Klontza D, Lagos P, et al. Age of pubertal stages including menarche in Greek girls. *Ann Hum Biol.* 1983;10:557–563
14. Lee MM, Chang KS, Chan MM. Sexual maturation of Chinese girls in Hong Kong. *Pediatrics.* 1963;32:389–398
15. Harlan WR, Harlan EA, Grillo GP. Secondary sex characteristics of girls 12 to 17 years of age: the U.S. Health Examination Survey. *J Pediatr.* 1980;96:1074–1078
16. Largo RH, Prader A. Pubertal development in girls. Variability and interrelationships. *Pediatrician.* 1987;14:212–218
17. Stratz CH. *Der Körper des kindes und seine pflege.* 3rd ed. Stuttgart, Germany: Enke; 1909
18. Reynolds EL, Wines JV. Individual differences of physical changes associated with adolescence in girls. *Am J Dis Child.* 1948;75:329–350
19. Prader A. Testicular size: assessment and clinical importance. *Triangle.* 1966;7:240–243
20. Tanner JM. The development of the reproductive system. In: *Growth at Adolescence.* Oxford, United Kingdom: Blackwell Scientific Publications; 1955

References, *continued*

21. Reynolds EL, Wines JV. Individual differences in physical changes associated with adolescence in boys. *Am J Dis Child.* 1951;82:529–547
22. Schonfeld WA, Beebe GW. Normal growth and variation in the male genitalia from birth to maturity. *J Urol.* 1942;48:759–777
23. Harries ML, Walker JM, Williams DM, Hawkins S, Hughes IA. Changes in the male voice at puberty. *Arch Dis Child.* 1997;77:445–447
24. Smithard A, Glazebrook C, Williams HC. Acne prevalence, knowledge about acne and psychological morbidity in mid-adolescence: a community-based study. *Br J Dermatol.* 2001;145:274–279
25. Burke BM, Cunliffe WJ. The assessment of acne vulgaris—the Leeds technique. *Br J Dermatol.* 1984;111:83–92
26. Largo RH, Prader A. Pubertal development in Swiss boys. *Helv Paediatr Acta.* 1983;38:211–228
27. Mul D, Fredriks AM, van Buuren S, Oostdük W, Verloove-Vanhorick SP, Wit JM. Pubertal development in The Netherlands 1965–1997. *Pediatr Res.* 2001;50:479–486